FOGSI
Medical Disorders in Pregnancy

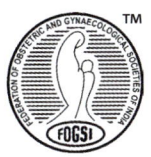
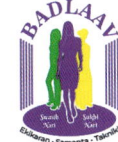

FOGSI
Medical Disorders in Pregnancy

Series Editor
Hrishikesh D Pai

Editors

Manoj Chellani MBBS DGO
Director
Aayush Hospital and Test Tube Baby Center
Raipur, Chhattisgarh, India
Chairperson, Medical Disorders in
Pregnancy Committee, FOGSI

Hrishikesh D Pai
MD FRCOG (UK-HON) FCPS FICOG MSc (USA)
President, FOGSI (Federation of Obstetric and
Gynaecological Societies of India)
Professor of Reproductive Medicine
D Y Patil University Navi Mumbai
Founder and Medical Director, Bloom IVF Group
Consultant Gynecologist
Lilavati Hospital IVF Center Mumbai
Consultant Gynecologist, Fortis Hospital Bloom
IVF Centre Delhi and Chandigarh, Mumbai,
Maharashtra, India

Yashodhara Pradeep
MD FICOG FICMCH FIUMB
Professor RLMCH Lucknow
Vice President FOGSI
Lucknow, Uttar Pradesh, India

Parikshit Tank
MD DNB FCPS DGO DFP MNAMS FICOG FRCOG
Consultant, Ashwini Maternity and Surgical
Hospital, Center for Endoscopy and ART
Mumbai, Maharashtra, India

Niranjan Chavan
MD FCPS FICOG DICOG MICOG DGO DFP
Diploma in Endoscopy (USA)
Professor
(Full) and Unit Chief
LTMMC and LTMG Hospital,
Mumbai, Maharashtra, India

Co-Editor

Neema Acharya MBBS DNB PhD
Professor and Head
Department of Obstetrics and Gynecology
Jawaharlal Nehru Medical College
Datta Meghe Institute of Higher Education and Research Wardha, Maharashtra, India

Foreword
Hrishikesh D Pai

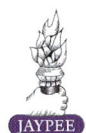

JAYPEE BROTHERS MEDICAL PUBLISHERS
The Health Sciences Publisher
New Delhi | London

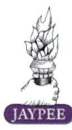 **Jaypee Brothers Medical Publishers (P) Ltd**

Headquarters
Jaypee Brothers Medical Publishers (P) Ltd
EMCA House, 23/23-B
Ansari Road, Daryaganj
New Delhi 110 002, India
Landline: +91-11-23272143, +91-11-23272703
+91-11-23282021, +91-11-23245672
Email: jaypee@jaypeebrothers.com

Corporate Office
Jaypee Brothers Medical Publishers (P) Ltd
4838/24, Ansari Road, Daryaganj
New Delhi 110 002, India
Phone: +91-11-43574357
Fax: +91-11-43574314
Email: jaypee@jaypeebrothers.com

Overseas Office
JP Medical Ltd.
83, Victoria Street, London
SW1H 0HW (UK)
Phone: +44 20 3170 8910
Fax: +44 (0)20 3008 6180
Email: info@jpmedpub.com

Website: www.jaypeebrothers.com
Website: www.jaypeedigital.com

© 2024, Jaypee Brothers Medical Publishers

The views and opinions expressed in this book are solely those of the original contributor(s)/author(s) and do not necessarily represent those of editor(s) or publisher of the book.

All rights reserved. No part of this publication may be reproduced, stored or transmitted in any form or by any means, electronic, mechanical, photocopying, recording or otherwise, without the prior permission in writing of the publishers.

All brand names and product names used in this book are trade names, service marks, trademarks or registered trademarks of their respective owners. The publisher is not associated with any product or vendor mentioned in this book.

Medical knowledge and practice change constantly. This book is designed to provide accurate, authoritative information about the subject matter in question. However, readers are advised to check the most current information available on procedures included and check information from the manufacturer of each product to be administered, to verify the recommended dose, formula, method and duration of administration, adverse effects and contra-indications. It is the responsibility of the practitioner to take all appropriate safety precautions. Neither the publisher nor the author(s)/editor(s) assume any liability for any injury and/or damage to persons or property arising from or related to use of material in this book.

This book is sold on the understanding that the publisher is not engaged in providing professional medical services. If such advice or services are required, the services of a competent medical professional should be sought.

Every effort has been made where necessary to contact holders of copyright to obtain permission to reproduce copyright material. If any have been inadvertently overlooked, the publisher will be pleased to make the necessary arrangements at the first opportunity.

Inquiries for bulk sales may be solicited at: jaypee@jaypeebrothers.com

FOGSI Medical Disorders in Pregnancy

First Edition: **2024**

ISBN: 978-93-5696-263-7

Printed at: Samrat Offset Pvt. Ltd.

Contributors

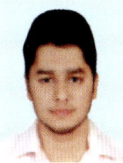

Ajay Adhikari MD (Medicine)
Senior Resident
Department of Medicine
RD Gardi Medical College
Ujjain, Madhya Pradesh, India

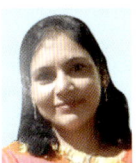

Archana Singh
MBBS DGO DNB FICOG
Professor
Government Medical College
Siddipet, Telangana, India
Vice President OGSH, Hyderabad

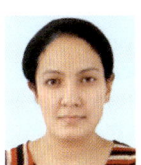

Devyani Misra
MBBS MD (Obs/Gyne) MRCOG (Lucknow)
Associate Professor
Dr Ram Manohar Lohia Institute of
Medical Sciences
Lucknow, Uttar Pradesh, India

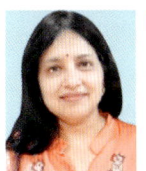

Divya Agrawal
MBBS MS FICOG FIAMS
Director
Ayushman Multispecialty Hospital
and Morpheus Aakriti IVF Centre
Varanasi, Uttar Pradesh, India

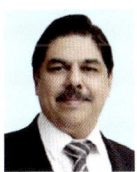

Hrishikesh D Pai
MD FRCOG (UK-HON) FCPS FICOG MSc
(USA)
President, FOGSI (Federation of
Obstetric and Gynaecological
Societies of India)
Professor of Reproductive Medicine
D Y Patil University Navi Mumbai
Founder and Medical Director
Bloom IVF Group Consultant
Gynecologist
Lilavati Hospital IVF Center Mumbai
Consultant Gynecologist, Fortis
Hospital Bloom IVF Centre
Delhi and Chandigarh, Mumbai,
Maharashtra, India

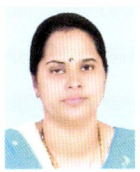

Indira Palo MBBS MD (Obs/Gyne)
Associate Professor
Department of Obstetrics and
Gynecology
MKCG Medical College and Hospital
Ganjam, Odisha, India

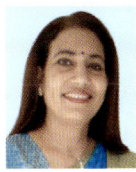

Jyoti Jaiswal MBBS MD (Obs/Gyne)
Professor and Head
Department of Obstetrics and
Gynecology
Pt JNM Medical College
Raipur, Chhattisgarh, India

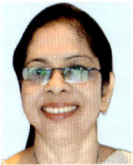

Jyoti Ramesh Chandran
MS FICOG Dip Urogynae
Professor and Head
Government Medical College
Kozhikode, Kerala, India

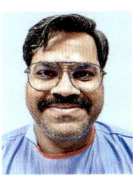

Lakshit Tomar MS (Surgery)
Senior Resident (Surgical Gastro)
Department of Surgical
Gastroenterology
Indira Gandhi Institute of Medical
Sciences
Patna, Bihar, India

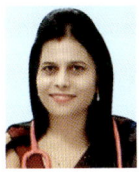

Mamta MBBS MS FMAS
Associate Professor
Department of Obstetrics
and Gynecology
Institute of Medical Sciences
Banaras Hindu University
Varanasi, Uttar Pradesh, India

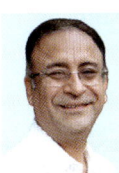

Manoj Chellani MBBS DGO
Director
Aayush Hospital and Test Tube
Baby Center
Raipur, Chhattisgarh, India
Chairperson, Medical Disorders in
Pregnancy Committee, FOGSI

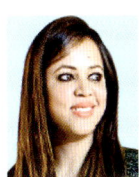

Mariyam Faruqi MBBS MS (Obs/Gyne)
Former Senior Resident
Department of Obstetrics
and Gynecology
Dr Ram Manohar Lohia Institute of
Medical Sciences
Lucknow, Uttar Pradesh, India

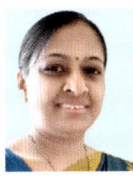

Neelamma Patil
MBBS MS (Obs/Gyne) FICOG
Professor
Department of Obstetrics and
Gynecology BLDE (D)
Shri BM Patil Medical College
Hospital and Research Center
Vijayapura, Karnataka, India

Contributors

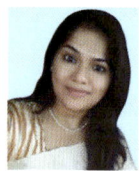

Neema Acharya MBBS DNB PhD
Professor and Head
Department of Obstetrics and
Gynecology
Jawaharlal Nehru Medical College
Datta Meghe Institute of Higher
Education and Research
Wardha, Maharashtra, India

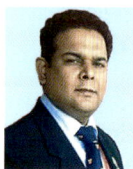

Niranjan Chavan
MD FCPS FICOG DICOG MICOG DGO DFP
Diploma in Endoscopy (USA)
Professor
(Full) and Unit Chief, LTMMC and
LTMG Hospital,
Mumbai, Maharashtra, India

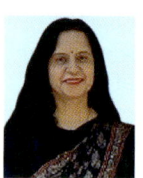

Padma Shukla MS FICOG FICMCH
Associate Professor
Department of Obstetrics and
Gynecology
Shyam Shah Medical College
Rewa, Madhya Pradesh, India

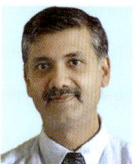

Parikshit Tank
MD DNB FCPS DGO DFP MNAMS FICOG
FRCOG
Consultant, Ashwini Maternity
and Surgical Hospital, Center for
Endoscopy and ART
Mumbai, Maharashtra, India

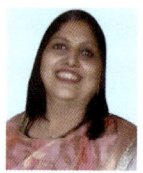

Pawan Preet Mann Gill
MBBS MS (Obs/Gyne)
Senior Consultant
Amrit Hospital
Rudrapur, Uttarakhand, India
Secretary, ROGS

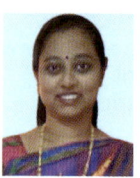

Rajasri G Yaliwal
MBBS MS (Obs/Gyne) FICOG
Professor
Department of Obstetrics and
Gynecology BLDE (D)
Shri BM Patil Medical College
Hospital and Research Center
Vijayapura, Karnataka, India

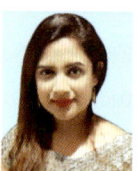

Revati Nitin Rane
MBBS DGO FCPS DNB
Director
Apex Multispecialty Hospital and
Akluj IVF and Test Tube Baby Center
Solapur, Maharashtra, India

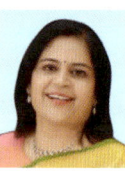

Richa Sharma DGO FICOG FMAS
Consultant
Pushpa Mission Hospital
Ujjain, Uttar Pradesh, India

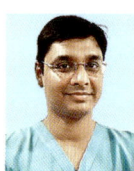

Saket Kumar
MS MCh (Surgical Gastro) FACS
Additional Professor
Department of Surgical
Gastroenterology
Indira Gandhi Institute of Medical
Sciences
Patna, Bihar, India

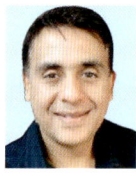

Samarth Shukla MBBS MD DNB PhD
Professor
Department of Pathology
Jawaharlal Nehru Medical College
Datta Meghe Institute of Higher
Education and Research
Wardha, Maharashtra, India

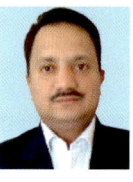

Sangamesh B Bhagavati
MBBS MD (General Medicine)
DM (Neurology)
Associate Professor
Department of General Medicine
BLDE (D)
Shri BM Patil Medical College
Hospital and Research Center
Vijayapura, Karnataka, India

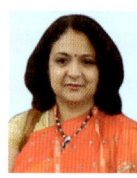

Shweta Kumari
MBBS (RIMS) DNB (Obs/Gyne) FICOG
Consultant Gynecologist
Sri Sathya Sai Sanjeevani Hospital
Jamshedpur, Jharkhand, India
Secretary, Jamshedpur Obstetrics
and Gynaecological Society

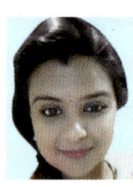

Sonal Agrawal MBBS MD
Assistant Professor
Department of Obstetrics and
Gynecology
Shyam Shah Medical College
Rewa, Madhya Pradesh, India

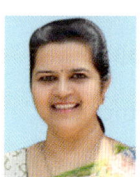

Sonal Gupta MBBS MD
Director and Head
Department of Obstetrics and
Gynecology
National Institute of Medical Sciences
Faridabad, Haryana, India

Contributors

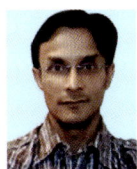

Sourya Acharya MBBS DNB PhD
Professor and Head
Department of Medicine
Jawaharlal Nehru Medical College
Datta Meghe Institute of Higher
Education and Research
Wardha, Maharashtra, India

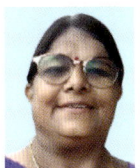

Sudesh Agrawal
MD (Obs/Gyne) DGES FICOG FICMCH
Gold Medalist
Senior Professor, Former Head and
Superintendent
Sardar Patel Medical College
Bikaner, Rajasthan, India

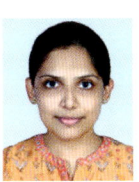

Supriya Gupta MBBS MS
DrNB SS (Gynecology Oncology)
Assistant Professor
Department of Obstetrics and
Gynecology
Pt JNM Medical College
Raipur, Chhattisgarh, India

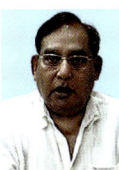

Vijay Prakash Singh
MD DNB MRCP (UK)
Professor
Department of Medical
Gastroenterology
Patna Medical College and
Hospital
Patna, Bihar, India

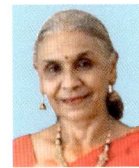

Yashodhara Pradeep
MD FICOG FICMCH FIUMB
Professor RLMCH Lucknow
Vice President FOGSI
Lucknow, Uttar Pradesh, India

Foreword

Dear all,

It gives me immense pleasure to present to you this book on *Medical Disorders in Pregnancy*. The book is a crisp compilation of chapters on all clinically relevant topics by none other than stalwarts in this field from all across the country.

Another highlight of this issue is that each of the contributing authors is a master of the topic they have contributed; these chapters are therefore rich with not only the recent evidence but also the vast experiences of the author, hence are full of practical tips and points, which the readers will find extremely beneficial.

FOGSI has always played a vital role in spreading the knowledge both among the doctors and the patients. This year my FOGSI slogan is *Swasthya Nari, Sukhi Nari*. My CSR activity is defined as *Badlaav* (Change) including three arms—*Ekikaran* (Integration of Thought and Action), *Samanta* (Equality of Treatment Irrespective of Economic Status), and *Takniki* (Technology to Achieve these Objectives). These books are a step toward my goal of improving women's health in our country, by providing updated information about the relevant topics in women care.

It will be a ready reckoner for both the students and the clinicians to update their knowledge on evidence-based management. I congratulate Dr Manoj Chellani, Chairperson, Medical Disorder in Pregnancy Committee; and all the Editors and Co-editors for their sincere efforts to write, collate, edit, and publish this book.

I sincerely hope that this book will benefit and empower all the FOGSIans. Wish you all a happy reading.

Hrishikesh D Pai
President, FOGSI (2022–2023)

Preface

It gives us great pride to present this book—*Medical Disorders in Pregnancy*. A textbook that will comprehensively, yet in a concise manner, covers all the quotidian topics under the umbrella of *Medical Disorders in Pregnancy*.

Medical science has seen accelerations by leaps and bounds in the last few decades and given us extensive knowledge of various conditions and their management. We as practitioners in the ever-evolving era need to keep pace with updates in the mundane yet important topics of obstetrics.

This textbook, a labor of love, aims at providing relevant literature to extract the most current evidence-based practices and then presenting them with concise, focused text, and crystal-clear clinical paradigms. This book is a small endeavor to give the latest information on various aspects of *Medical Disorders in Pregnancy*, which will be of great help to obstetricians. Each chapter discusses the clinical problems, differential diagnosis, diagnostic work-up, and various recent treatment modalities, which could improve the care of the patients.

This book incorporates the most common disorders of pregnancy encompassing topics such as anemia and hypertensive disorders of pregnancy. It also mentions various endocrinal disorders such as diabetes, thyroid-related disorders, and the raising issue of obesity. It includes topics related to systemic disorders pertaining to central nervous system (CNS) such as epilepsy; cardiovascular system (CVS) such as heart diseases, liver, and renal diseases. Some highlights about Rh-isoimmunization and systemic lupus erythematosus (SLE) are also explained. The book contains information on infections such as human immunodeficiency virus (HIV), hepatitis, urinary tract infection (UTI), dengue, and also the recent pandemic with lack of literature, which the world was exposed to COVID.

We are sincerely thankful to the other contributors, which include leading clinicians and academicians from the length and breadth of the country. They have put in their best efforts to give recent updates and future possible developments.

Manoj Chellani
Hrishikesh D Pai
Yashodhara Pradeep
Parikshit Tank
Niranjan Chavan

Contents

1. **Anemia in Pregnancy** 1
   Archana Singh

2. **Hypertensive Disorders of Pregnancy** 8
   Jyoti Ramesh Chandran

3. **Diabetes in Pregnancy** 16
   Pawan Preet Mann Gill

4. **Obesity in Pregnancy** 28
   Revati Nitin Rane

5. **Thyroid Disorders in Pregnancy** 37
   Neema Acharya, Sourya Acharya, Samarth Shukla

6. **Asthma in Pregnancy** 42
   Jyoti Jaiswal, Supriya Gupta

7. **Heart Diseases in Pregnancy** 50
   Divya Agrawal

8. **Liver Diseases in Pregnancy** 64
   Shweta Kumari

9. **Renal Disorders in Pregnancy** 72
   Manoj Chellani

10. **Epilepsy in Pregnancy** 83
    Rajasri G Yaliwal, Neelamma Patil, Sangamesh B Bhagavati

11. **Rh Alloimmunization** 89
    Mariyam Faruqi, Devyani Misra

12. **Systemic Lupus Erythematosus in Pregnancy** 99
    Sonal Gupta

13. **Hepatitis B Infection in Pregnancy** 108
    Padma Shukla, Sonal Agrawal

14. **Urinary Tract Infection in Pregnancy** 113
    Mamta

15. **Dengue in Pregnancy** 118
    Richa Sharma, Ajay Adhikari

16. HIV in Pregnancy 125
Indira Palo

17. SARS-CoV-2 during Pregnancy 133
Sudesh Agrawal

18. Pregnancy-related Constipation 143
Saket Kumar, Lakshit Tomar, Vijay Prakash Singh

Index *149*

Chapter 1

Anemia in Pregnancy

Archana Singh

■ INTRODUCTION

A third of the world's population suffers from anemia, a disorder marked by low levels of hemoglobin (Hb). The most frequent medical condition that complicates pregnancy is anemia, which is more prevalent in developing nations. For the purpose of creating successful interventions and avoiding consequences, understanding anemia is essential.

■ DEFINITION OF ANEMIA

Anemia is a blood disorder in which there are fewer red blood cells (RBCs) than usual or less Hb in the blood, which leads to reduced ability of the blood to carry oxygen that is insufficient to meet physiologic needs. While the World Health Organization (WHO) defines anemia in pregnancy as Hb values <11 g/dL,[2] the Centre for Disease Control and Prevention (CDC) define anemia in pregnancy as Hb <11 g/dL [hematocrit (HCT); 33%] in the first and third trimesters and <10.5 g/dL (HCT; 32%) in the second trimester. According to the WHO, anemia in postpartum females is Hb <10 g/dL.[2]

Anemia is defined as having the following Hb and HCT levels:
- First trimester:[7] Hb <11 g/dL; HCT <33%
- Second trimester: Hb <10.5 g/dL; HCT <32%
- Third trimester: Hb <11 g/dL; HCT <33%.

Anemia classification based on Hb levels:
- Mild anemia: 9–10.9 g/dL
- Moderate anemia: 7–8.9 g/dL
- Severe anemia: <7 g/dL
- Very severe anemia: <4 g/dL.

■ COMMON CAUSES OF ANEMIA IN PREGNANCY

- *Infections:* Urinary tract infection (UTI), hookworm, and malaria
- Acute or chronic hemorrhagic blood loss
- *Genetic/hemoglobinopathies:* Thalassemia, sickle cell disease (SCD), rare kinds include hemolytic leukemia, Hodgkin's disease, autoimmunity, paroxysmal nocturnal hemoglobinuria, aplastic anemia, renal illness, and bone marrow disorders.

Physiological Anemia

During pregnancy, erythroid hyperplasia of the marrow occurs, and RBC mass increases by 25% and plasma volume increases by 50%. Disproportionate increase in plasma volume results in hemodilution during pregnancy and Hb concentration naturally declines during the first and second trimesters, rising gradually again in the third trimester. Therefore, the HCT drops from between 38 and 45% as found in healthy women who are not pregnant to roughly 34% during late pregnancy. The oxygen-carrying capacity is constant during pregnancy despite hemodilution.

The following are some criteria for physiological anemia:
- Hb: 10 g/dL
- RBC: 3.2 million/mm^3
- Packed cell volume (PCV): 30
- Peripheral smear showing normal morphology of RBC with central pallor.

Thus, if Hb is <11.5 g/dL at the onset of pregnancy, women may be treated prophylactically because subsequent hemodilution usually reduces Hb to <10 g/dL.

Iron Requirement during Pregnancy

During pregnancy, the maternal total iron requirement is 1,000 mg.
- For maternal Hb mass growth 450 mg is needed.
- The placenta and fetus need 360 mg
- Replacement of daily loss from stools, skin, and urine need 200–250 mg of iron
- Replacement of lost blood during childbirth (150 to 200 mg).

Thus, the maternal demand for iron during pregnancy increases from 1–2 mg in the first trimester to 6–8 mg in the third trimester. Average 4 mg/day iron will be required by the woman.

Iron Deficiency Anemia

Iron deficiency affects about 95% of pregnant women with anemia.[5] Iron deficiency anemia (IDA) during pregnancy poses a number of maternal and fetal difficulties, including placental abnormalities, intrauterine growth retardation, preterm birth, and a decrease in infant iron storage, hence it is crucial to diagnose and treat the condition effectively. In addition to anemia symptoms, maternal problems can lead to low blood reserves during labor and delivery, significant blood loss that necessitates transfusion, cardiac stress, an extended hospital stay, decreased breast milk supply, and low iron reserves in the mother during and after delivery.

Etiology of Iron Deficiency Anemia

- Dietary iron deficiency
- Worm infestation
- Chronic menorrhagia
- Chronic infections
- Repeated pregnancies
- <1 year birth interval
- Multiple pregnancies.

Phases of Anemia

- *Prelatent (depletion):*
  - Stores are depleted without a change in HCT or serum iron levels
  - Reduced stored iron, serum ferritin with normal Hb
- *Latent (iron deficient erythropoiesis):*
  - Without a change in the HCT, serum iron decreases and the total iron-binding capacity (TIBC) rises
  - Reduced stored and transport iron
  - Increased erythrocyte protoporphyrin concentration detected by a routine transferrin saturation test (about 20–50%)
- *IDA:*
  - When a decline in HCT is accompanied by clinical features of anemia.

EFFECTS OF ANEMIA IN PREGNANCY

- *Mother:*
  - *Antepartum:* Poor weight gain, pre-eclampsia, infection, preterm labor, premature rupture of membrane (PROM), and high output cardiac failure
  - *Intrapartum:* Dysfunctional labor, hemorrhage, and cardiac failure

- *Postpartum:* Subinvolution of uterus; decreased lactation, puerperal sepsis, puerperal venous thrombosis, pulmonary embolism, and delayed general recovery after cesarean section
- *Fetus:*
  - Intrauterine growth restriction (IUGR)
  - Preterm birth
  - Low-birth-weight[6] (LBW)
  - Delayed cognitive function.

The HCT of newborns whose mothers have IDA is often normal, but they typically have reduced iron storage, an increased risk of IDA in the early months, and a need for early iron supplements.

CLINICAL FEATURES OF ANEMIA

Depending on the cause of the anemia, the severity of the onset and the presence of additional comorbidities, a patient may or may not experience anemia symptoms. Patients with moderate anemia may not show any symptoms, but when the Hb level falls below 7.0 g/dL, the majority of patients start to show anemia-related symptoms.

The most prevalent clinical symptoms of anemia, such as fatigue, low physical and mental capacity, weakness, headache loss of appetite, dry and cracked lips and brittle hair, dysphagia, paresthesia, giddiness, shortness of breath, palpitations, leg cramps, ankle swelling, and cold intolerance are explained by the critical role of Hb to carry oxygen to the tissues.

The main indicators of anemia are as follows:
- Conjunctival and palmar pallor
- Angular stomatitis
- Glossitis
- Skin that is dry or has a rough texture
- Increased jugular venous pressure (JVP)
- Heart murmurs
- Tachycardia
- Tachypnea
- Postural hypotension
- Koilonychia.

INVESTIGATIONS

- Diagnosis of anemia begins with complete blood count (CBC); usually, if women have anemia, subsequent testing is based on whether the mean corpuscular volume (MCV) is low (<79 fL) or high (>100 fL).
- *For microcytic anemias:* Evaluation includes testing for iron deficiency and hemoglobinopathies.
- *For macrocytic anemias:* Evaluation includes serum folate and vitamin B12 levels.
- *For anemia with mixed causes:* Evaluation for both types is required.
- In IDA, serum ferritin is the first to become abnormal. In patients without underlying inflammation, measuring serum ferritin levels is the most accurate test.
- Plasma ferritin concentrations range from 15 to 300 ng/mL.
- Since serum ferritin is an acute phase reactant, it may be normal or even high under inflammatory conditions even when anemia is present. In these circumstances, further testing may be necessary to confirm the diagnosis.
- Serum iron concentration (<12 µmol/L)
- Low transferrin saturation (350 mg/dL) and increase in TIBC (>400 µg/dL)
- Increased serum soluble transferrin binding receptors (>8 mg/L)
- Examinations of the urine, serum protein, and stools for ova, cysts, and hidden blood, aid in the diagnosis and treatment of IDA.
- Other procedures used to assess unexplained anemia include free erythrocyte porphyrin, Hb electrophoresis, and bone marrow examination.

PREVENTION OF IRON DEFICIENCY

- The Cochrane database states that routine iron or iron and folate supplementation does prevent low maternal Hb at delivery. In places where the prevalence of iron insufficiency is <40%, the WHO advises universal oral iron supplementation with 60 mg of elemental iron daily for 6 months during pregnancy. In areas where the prevalence is >40%, the recommendation is to continue supplementation for 3 months postpartum.
- The American College of Obstetricians and Gynecologists and the CDC both advise supplementing with 30 mg of elemental iron daily. The choice of universal or selective prophylaxis depends on the prevalence of iron deficiency in the obstetric population served as well as nutritional, economic, and social factors.[3]
- Ministry of health, Government of India, recommendation for iron in pregnancy is 100 mg of elemental iron with 500 μg of folic acid in second half of pregnancy for at least 100 days.[1]

MANAGEMENT

Objectives
- To treat anemia and achieve a normal Hb level by the end of pregnancy.
- To replenish iron stores by parenteral or oral iron supplementation and blood transfusion.

Three primary considerations determine the choice of method:
1. Severity of the anemia
2. Gestational age
3. Assessment of additional risk factor.

Dietary Advice

Iron absorption depends upon the amount of iron in diet as well as its bioavailability

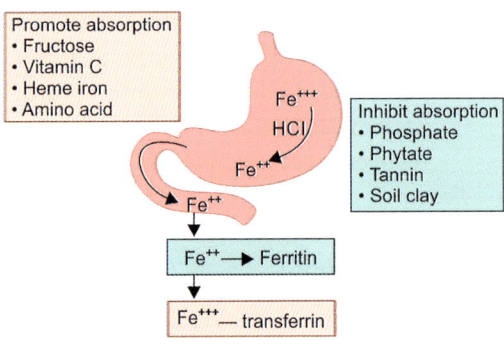

Iron absorption.

and physiological requirements. The most accessible type of iron in the diet is heme iron (5%), which is found in foods such as animal meat, viscera, and blood, while non-heme iron is found in cereals, vegetables, milk, and eggs, and accounts for the other 95%. Nonheme iron absorption is boosted by ascorbic acid and proteins, and blocked by phytates, calcium, tea, and coffee. Consuming foods high in vitamin C and germinated legumes can also increase iron absorption. Therefore, all pregnant women should get dietary counseling, including information on sources of food high in iron, elements that may encourage or impede absorption, and the significance of keeping appropriate iron levels.[3]

Treatment to Reverse the Anemia

Treatment for anemia during pregnancy aims to reverse the anemia. Serum ferritin should be measured at least once early in pregnancy. If ferritin and Hb levels are normal, preventive oral iron therapy should be started. If ferritin and Hb levels indicate iron deficiency, anemia treatment should be started. Later in pregnancy, serum ferritin does not need to be remeasured unless anemic symptoms appear. On the other hand, Hb should be assessed every trimester because there is always a chance that the body will require more iron and develop an iron shortage.[4]

Oral Iron Therapy

Oral iron should be the preferred first-line treatment for iron deficiency.[5]

For prevention 30–60 mg of elemental iron and 400 g of folic acid (WHO 2021) and for a woman diagnosed with anemia elemental iron should be increased to 120 mg.

60 mg of elemental iron is 300 mg of Ferrous sulfate/180 mg of ferrous fumarate or 500 mg of ferrous gluconate.

Ferrous sulfate 325 mg orally once a day is usually effective [Royal College of Obstetricians and Gynaecologists (RCOG)].

Higher or more frequent doses increase gastrointestinal (GI) adverse effects, especially constipation, and one dose blocks absorption of the next dose, thereby reducing percentage intake.

Other formulations may contain either the bivalent ferrous form or the trivalent ferric form. Compared to trivalent formulations, bivalent ferrous iron preparations are more easily absorbed; however, they are also more likely to cause side effects such as nausea, vomiting, diarrhea, constipation, and abdominal pain.

Drawbacks

- Unpredictable absorption rate and intolerance are some of the drawbacks. It is not suitable for patients with GI problems and noncompliant patients.
- Needs long time for improvement.

The response to treatment of elemental iron is rapid and can be assessed by improvement in general wellbeing of patient, rise of Hb by 0.8 g/dL/week and increase in reticulocyte count. Within 5–10 days of starting treatment, the reticulocyte count rises. The presence of concurrent folate insufficiency should be suspected if iron supplements are ineffective. If there is no clinical or hematologic response after 3–4 weeks of oral iron therapy, diagnostic reevaluation is needed.

Parenteral Iron Therapy

About 20% of expectant women cannot absorb enough oral iron supplements. When oral iron is not accepted or absorbed, and when patient compliance is in question, or when a woman is getting close to term and there is not enough time (6–8 weeks before delivery) for oral supplementation to be successful, parenteral iron is advised (RCOG, Level evidence C).

Parenteral iron can be infused intravenously or given intramuscularly. Among the parenteral forms of iron are ferric carboxymaltose, ferric sucrose, and iron dextran.

The Ganzoni formula [total iron dose = {Body weight × (15 − actual Hb)} × 2.4 + iron storage] may be used to determine the iron shortfall.

Intramuscular Route

Iron dextran (1 mL contains 50 mg elemental iron and 1 amp = 2 mL)

Dose: 100 mg intramuscular (IM) once daily.

Drawbacks: It is painful injection and can cause skin discoloration, local abscess, and allergic reactions.

Iron Sucrose Complex

Each mL of iron hydroxide sucrose complex contains 20 mg of iron and is given as intravenous infusion after dilution with 100 mL of normal saline. After intravenous administration it dissociates into iron and sucrose. In 7–14 days, a noticeable increase in reticulocyte count is expected.

Advantages of iron sucrose over others:
- All iron preparations can cause tissue peroxidation except iron sucrose
- Less risk of tissue parenchymal injury by free iron
- Safe for people with dextran sensitivity
- Minimal side effects
- The Hb rise will be evident in as early as 5 days.

Disadvantage: Needs a set up where anaphylactic reaction can be managed.

Ferric Carboxymaltose is a new compound which does not require test dose to be administered and can be given by bolus intravenous injection or a fast intravenous infusion. However, due to the lack of human data on the effects of pregnancy, it can only be used to treat anemia in postpartum patients.

Blood Transfusion

The decision for blood transfusion should not be based only on HCT. Blood transfusion is indicated for anemia with severe constitutional or cardiopulmonary signs and symptoms and risk of developing complications of inadequate oxygenation.

Indications for blood transfusion include:
- Severe anemia, particularly after 36 weeks
- Risk of further hemorrhage
- Concurrent infections
- Imminent cardiac compromise.

Management During Labor
- Delivery should be planned in well-equipped hospital with facilities for blood transfusion.
- During labor, pain management should be taken into account, as should oxygen therapy.
- Prophylactic forceps/vacuum to cut short second stage labor.
- Third stage of labor must be actively managed to reduce blood loss.

If a woman has anemia caused by iron deficiency, she should continue taking oral supplements for at least 3 months.

Folate Deficiency

Folates are necessary for the development of the fetal nervous system, RBC maturation, and the synthesis of purines and pyrimidines. It is plentiful in various plant foods, and meats, particularly raw green leafy vegetables, fruits, and organ meats. The bioavailability of folate is higher when it is present in supplements or fortified foods than when it naturally occurs in food because prolonged cooking destroys it.

Etiology of Folate Deficiency Anemia
- Inadequate intake—nutritional deficiency or alcohol
- Increased demand (e.g., due to pregnancy or lactation)
- Reduction in absorption (due to certain drugs).

Folate insufficiency can also be caused by inadequate absorption and excessive excretion. Insufficient folate during pregnancy raises the chance of neural tube abnormalities in addition to causing anemia. Testing in the laboratory is necessary to confirm the diagnosis. Megaloblastic anemia serum with serum folate <3 µg/L, helps in the diagnosis. Measurement of neutrophil hyper segmentation is sensitive and readily available.

The recommended daily allowance (RDA) of folate for pregnant women is 400 µg per day. 4,000 µg/day is the suggested dose for women who have previously given birth to a child with a neural tube defect, and it should be started at least 1 month prior to conception.

Outcomes and treatments for other forms of inherited and acquired anemia in pregnancy vary by disease, and include nutritional supplementation, corticosteroids, supportive transfusions, and splenectomy.

■ REFERENCES

1. Ministry of Health and Family Welfare. Guidelines for Control of Iron Deficiency Anaemia. Government of India: Ministry of Health and Family Welfare; 2013.
2. World Health Organization. Assessing, preventing, and controlling iron deficiency anaemia. Geneva: World Health Organization; 2001.
3. Recommendations to prevent and control iron deficiency in the United States. Centers for Disease Control and Prevention. MMWR Recomm Rep. 1998;47(RR-3):1-29.
4. Tran K, McCormack S. Screening and Treatment of Obstetric Anemia: A Review of Clinical Effectiveness, Cost-Effectiveness, and Guidelines. Ottawa (ON): Canadian Agency for Drugs and Technologies in Health; 2019.
5. James AH. Iron Deficiency Anaemia in Pregnancy. Obstet Gynecol. 2021;138(4):663-674.
6. Montoya Romero Jde J, Castelazo Morales E, Valerio Castro E, Velázquez Cornejo G, Nava Muñoz DA, Escárcega Preciado JA, et al. Review by expert group in the diagnosis and treatment of anemia in pregnant women. Federación Mexicana de Colegios de Obstetricia y Ginecología. Ginecol Obstet Mex. 2012;80(9):563-80.
7. C Breymann; Anaemia Working Group. Current aspects of diagnosis and treatment of iron deficiency anemia in pregnancy. Praxis (Bern 1994). 2001;90(31-32):1283-91.

Chapter 2
Hypertensive Disorders of Pregnancy

Jyoti Ramesh Chandran

■ INTRODUCTION

Hypertensive disorders of pregnancy (HDP) remain a major cause of maternal and perinatal morbidity and mortality despite advances in diagnosis and treatment. Preeclampsia (PE) accounts for over 500,000 fetal and neonatal deaths and over 70,000 maternal deaths globally every year.

A systolic blood pressure (SBP) of ≥140 mm Hg and/or a diastolic blood pressure (DBP) of ≥90 mm Hg are indicative of hypertension in pregnancy. The BP should be confirmed by repeated measurements over few hours or repeated after 15 minutes if a SBP of ≥160 mm Hg and/or DBP of ≥110 mm Hg is detected.[1]

Classification of HDP (Box 1)

BOX 1: International Society for Study of Hypertension in Pregnancy (ISSHP) classification.

Hypertension known before pregnancy or hypertension that presents in first 20 weeks of pregnancy
- Chronic hypertension
  - Essential hypertension
  - Secondary hypertension
- White coat hypertension
- Masked hypertension

Hypertension arising de novo or at or after 20 weeks of pregnancy
- Transient gestational hypertension
- Gestational hypertension
- Preeclampsia-de novo or superimposed on chronic hypertension

Important differences from previous classification:
- Proteinuria is no longer mandatory for diagnosis of PE.
- PE is not graded from mild to severe, instead nonsevere and severe PE and early-onset preeclampsia (EOPE) if it is detected before 34 weeks of pregnancy and late-onset preeclampsia (LOPE) if detected after 34 weeks of gestation.
- The hemolysis, elevated liver enzymes, and low platelet count) (HELLP) syndrome is a serious manifestation of PE and not considered a separate disorder.

■ PREECLAMPSIA (TABLES 1 AND 2)

- PE is a disorder of pregnancy associated with new-onset hypertension, which occurs most often after 20 weeks of gestation and frequently near term

TABLE 1: Risk factors for preeclampsia.

- Nulliparity
- Multifetal gestation
- Preeclampsia in previous pregnancy
- Chronic hypertension
- Pregestational diabetes
- Gestational diabetes
- Thrombophilia
- Systemic lupus erythematosus
- Prepregnancy body mass index >30
- Antiphospholipid antibody syndrome
- Maternal age 35 years or older
- Kidney disease
- Assisted reproductive technology
- Obstructive sleep apnea

TABLE 2: Classification of preeclampsia (PE) (ACOG 2013).

	Nonsevere PE	Severe PE
Blood pressure	≥140/90 but <160/110 mm Hg	≥160/110 mm Hg
Symptoms	Absence of headache, visual symptoms, pulmonary edema, oliguria	Presence of headache, visual symptoms pulmonary edema, oliguria (Urine output <400 mL/24 hours)
Investigations	Laboratory investigations for PE are normal	• Thrombocytopenia (platelet ≤100,000 mm^3), elevated liver enzymes (AST/ALT > twice normal) • Elevated serum creatinine (<1.1 mg/dL)
Proteinuria (Exclude by ACOG 2013)	≤2 + on dipstick	>2 + on dipstick (or) >5 g/24 hours
Fetal status (exclude by ACOG 2013)	No fetal growth restriction	Fetal growth restriction may be present

(ACOG: American College of Obstetricians and Gynecologists; ALT: alanine transaminase; AST: aspartate transaminase)

- EOP occurs ≤34 weeks
- LOP occurs ≥34 weeks.

PATHOGENESIS OF PREECLAMPSIA

Early-onset Preeclampsia

Absence of placental remodelling plays a major role in pathogenesis of preeclampsia **(Table 3)**. Early-onset preeclampsia (<34 weeks) is usually due to angiogenic imbalance, e.g., soluble fms-like tyrosine kinase-1 (sFlt-1) and soluble endoglins are increased and reduction in proangiogenic factors, e.g., placental growth factor (PlGF). It is primary placental under perfusion-related PE dangerous to the women. It is predominate in low-income countries. Seen as shorter time between first intercourse, coitarche, and first pregnancy, thereby reducing opportunity for exposure to paternal antigen through exposure to seminal fluid; this reduces maternal immune adaptiveness that facilitates normal placental development

Late-onset Preeclampsia

According to the Screening for Pregnancy Endpoints Consortium (SCOPE) study, it is maternal response to pregnancy and is related to factors that predict later cardiovascular disease though metabolic syndrome. It is associated with obesity-proinflammatory state and may be amplified by burden of infectious diseases and chronic inflammation.

TABLE 3: Placental remodelling.

Placental changes in normal pregnancy	Placental changes in preeclampsia
• Tumor like extra-villous trophoblast invade maternal spiral arteries • Become endovascular trophoblast partially replacing maternal endothelium • Hybrid vessel lined by maternal and fetal cells	• Inadequate invasion by extravillous trophoblast • Absent or deficient remodeling of the spiral arteries necessary for adequate placental perfusion. • Vasospasm + vascular occlusion • Reduced placental perfusion

AREAS OF RESEARCH SHOWING EVIDENCES

Why not all women with reduced placental perfusion have PE? Moreover, reduced placental perfusion also occurs in fetal growth restriction (FGR) and preterm labor. Perhaps, reduced placental perfusion must interact with maternal risk factors. Genetically inherited factors associated with endothelial dysfunction are related to immune cytotrophoblastic-mediated cytotrophoblastic cell invasion which may be due to defective human leukocyte antigen-G (HLA-G) expression, mother with AA genotype + fetus with HLA-C2 phenotype. Defective HLA-G expression contributes to inadequate trophoblastic invasion. Trophoblast become vulnerable to attack by placental natural killer (pNK) cells and their invasion is not facilitated by uterine natural killer (uNK) cells. NK may act as friends or foes depending on which population of NK cells are dominant.

Seminal priming also plays an important role. Paternal alloantigens play a pivotal role in embryonal cell interaction with maternal immune system

Endothelial cells regulate nutrient exchange, modulate inflammatory processes, and play primary role in angiogenesis. Endothelial function is affected in chronic hypertension, diabetes or insulin resistance (severity of hypertension and diabetes directly correlated with risk of developing PE), renal disease, dyslipidemia, various thrombophilias (antiphospholipid syndrome, protein C or S deficiency, antithrombin deficiency, and factor V Leiden mutation), urinary tract infection, and periodontal disease.

There are factors related to immune-mediated invasion and angiogenesis. These include primiparity, primipaternity, condom use [maternal major histocompatibility complex (MHC) class 1 and 2 and tolerance to paternal MHC 1 and 2 occurs after long exposure to paternal seminal fluid], intrauterine insemination (IUI) or in vitro fertilization (IVF) with donor gametes, twins, and molar pregnancy.

Oxidative Stress Hypothesis

Sera of woman with PE had markedly reduced antioxidant activity. Oxidative stress in placenta releases sFLT-1 [antagonizes angiogenic factors such as vascular endothelial growth factor (VEGF) and PlGF], soluble endoglin proinflammatory cytokine, and trophoblast debris leading to inflammatory milieu causes generalized endothelial dysfunction.

MECHANISM OF END-ORGAN DAMAGE IN PREECLAMPSIA

- Endothelial dysfunction leads to vasospasm which causes hypertension, oliguria, abruptio placentae, and seizure. Capillary leak causes edema, pulmonary edema, proteinuria, headache, blurring of vision, and epigastric pain.
- Activation of coagulation cascade leads to thrombocytopenia, hemorrhage, and disseminated intravascular coagulopathy increased cardiac afterload.
- *Cardiovascular changes:* Increased left ventricular mass, increased left-sided filling pressure, and extravasation of fluid into extracellular space (especially lungs).
- *Changes in blood parameters:* Hemoconcentration, hypovolemia, and thrombocytopenia.
- Evidence of intravascular coagulation [prolonged prothrombin time and activated partial thromboplastin time (APTT)] and erythrocyte destruction seen as elevated lactate dehydrogenase (LDH) levels.
- *Endocrine system:* Decreased renin, angiotensin 2, and aldosterone, increased deoxycorticosterone (cause of sodium retention), and normal vasopressin.
- *Fluid electrolyte levels:* Expanded extracellular fluid, electrolyte concentration not disturbed much but decreased pH and bicarbonates.
- *Kidneys:* Renal perfusion and glomerular filtration rate (GFR) decreases, serum creatinine and uric acid increases, and urinary calcium decreases

- *Liver:* Periportal hemorrhage, transaminase levels increase, and chances of hepatic rupture
- *Brain:* Type1 changes—hemorrhage, type 2 changes—edema, hyperemia, ischemia, and thrombosis.
- *Uteroplacental:* Microthrombosis in placenta, uteroplacental insufficiency, and Doppler changes in uterine arteries.

Drugs used in HDP **Table 4** and maternal and fetal complications in PE **Table 5**.

■ ECLAMPSIA

Convulsions occurring in a woman with PE (**Table 6**).

Incidence: Antepartum 50% (III TM), intrapartum 30%, and postpartum 20% (within 48 hours of delivery). Convulsions occurring beyond 7 days of delivery are unlikely due to eclampsia

Status Eclampticus

It is defined as occurrence of convulsions continuously without any seizure-free interval. Interval time is usually considered as 30 minutes. It can result in prolonged coma and death.

Intercurrent Eclampsia

It is defined as when pregnancy is continued for at least 2 days to 2 weeks following eclampsia. It is controversial as pregnancy is usually terminated within 24-48 hours in eclampsia due to high perinatal and maternal morbidity and mortality.

TABLE 4: Drugs used in pregnancy.

Drugs	Mechanism of action	Dosage	Side effects
Methyldopa	Central and peripheral antiadrenergic	• 250 mg BD up to 2 g/day PO • Effect appears after 48 hours	• Maternal: Postural HT, drowsiness, hemolytic anemia, and positive Coombs test • Fetal: Safe
Labetalol	• Alpha and beta adrenergic • Beta blocker	• 100 mg BD PO • Maximum 1,200/day • HT crisis: 20 mg IV bolus → 40–220 mg every 10 minutes	• Maternal: Flushing, hypotension • Fetal: Safe
Nifedipine	Calcium channel blocker	• 5 mg BD – 80 mg PO • HT crisis: 10 mg → 20 mg IV Bolus → 40 mg to 220 mg every 10 min	• Maternal: Flushing, hypotension, headache, tachycardia, palpitations • Fetal: Safe
Hydralazine	Peripheral arterial vasodilator	• HT crisis: 5–10 mg IV every 15 minutes • Maximum 30 mg	• Maternal: Flushing, hypotension, headache, tachycardia, palpitations, lupus-like syndrome • Fetal: Safe. Can cause fetal thrombocytopenia
Sodium nitroprusside	Direct arterial and venous vasodilator	0.3 µg/kg/min	• Maternal: Hypotension, vomiting • Fetal: Toxicity due to cyanide and thiocyanate
Nitroglycerine	Venous relaxation	5 µg/min IV	• Maternal: Headache, methemoglobinemia • CI in HT encephalopathy as it increases ICP

(HT: hypertension; ICP: intracranial pressure; IV: intravenous)

TABLE 5: Maternal and fetal complications in preeclampsia

Maternal complications			Fetal complications
Antepartum	*Intrapartum*	*Postpartum*	
• Eclampsia (50%) • Cerebral hemorrhage • Cortical blindness • Pulmonary oedema • Cardiac failiure • Liver hematoma • Abruptio placentae • HELLP Syndrome • Renal failure • DIC • Preterm Labour (Iatrogenic)	Eclampsia (30%)	• Eclampsia (20%) • Postpartum hemorrhage • Shock	• Fetal growth restriction • Birth asphyxia • Intrauterine fetal demise • Prematurity
Recurrence risk: Preeclampsia 25%		**Chronic hypertension 40%**	

TABLE 6: Description of convulsion in eclampsia.

Stage	Duration	Clinical features
Premonitory	30 seconds	Rolling up of eyeballs, twitching of limbs and face
Tonic stage	15–20 seconds	Generalized tonic contraction of the body, opisthotonus, cessation of respiration, clenching of hands, protrusion of tongue
Clonic stage	1 minute	Muscles of the body contract and relax, tongue bite occurs, secretions from mouth
Postictal stage	Few minutes	Patient in drowsy or confused state

Differential Diagnosis for Convulsions in Pregnancy

It includes eclampsia, epilepsy, meningitis, encephalitis, cortical venous thrombosis, metabolic abnormalities such as hypoglycemia and electrolyte imbalance, hypertensive encephalopathy, intracranial tumor, and neurocysticercosis. However, convulsions occurring during pregnancy and during 48 hours of delivery are assumed to be eclampsia until proved otherwise. Complications of eclampsia include intracranial hemorrhage, aspiration pneumonia, cardiopulmonary arrest, renal failure, abruption and disseminated intravascular coagulation (DIC), injuries—tongue bite, etc., and fetal hypoxia and death.

However, eclampsia may not be preceded by PE. Two randomized placebo-controlled trials indicate that seizure occurred in only a small proportion of patients with PE (1.9%) or severe PE (3.2%). It is also noteworthy that there are significant proportion of patients who had abrupt-onset eclampsia without warning signs or symptoms. In a nationwide analysis of cases of eclampsia in the United Kingdom, it was noted that in 38% of eclamptic cases the seizure occurred without any prior documentation of either hypertension or proteinuria in the hospital setting. Thus, the notion that PE has a natural linear progression from PE without severe features to PE with severe features and eventually to eclamptic convulsions is inaccurate. Two clinical entities which need mention are posterior reversible

TABLE 7: Hemolysis, elevated liver enzymes, and low platelet count (HELLP) syndrome.

Hemolysis	Elevated liver enzymes	Low platelets
Abnormal peripheral smear- presence of schistocytes and burr cells	Serum aspartate aminotransferase (AST) and alanine aminotransferase (ALT) >70 IU/L (more than twice normal)	<100,000/mm^3
Total bilirubin >1.2 mg/dL	LDH > 600 IU/L	
Low serum haptoglobin (<25 mg/dL)		
Lactate dehydrogenase (LDH) >600 IU/L		

encephalopathy syndrome (PRES) and reversible cerebral vasoconstriction syndrome (RCVS).

The PRES is a constellation of a range of clinical neurologic signs and symptoms such as vision loss or deficit, seizure, headache, and altered sensorium or confusion. Although suspicion for PRES is increased in the setting of these clinical features, the diagnosis of PRES is made by the presence of vasogenic edema and hyperintensities in the posterior aspects of the brain on magnetic resonance imaging (MRI).

Women are particularly at risk of PRES in the settings of eclampsia and PE with headache, altered consciousness, or visual abnormalities. RVCS on the other hand is characterized by reversible multifocal narrowing of the arteries of the brain with signs and symptoms that typically include thunderclap headache and, less commonly, focal neurologic deficits related to brain edema, stroke, or seizure. Treatment of women with PRES and RVCS may include medical control of hypertension, antiepileptic medication, and long-term neurologic follow-up.

Pathogenesis includes generalized vasospasm and endothelial damage leads to activation of coagulation cascade, platelet aggregation, and end-organ damage. Complete HELLP if all three components are seen. Partial HELLP if one or two components are there **(Table 7)**.

Chronic Hypertension in Pregnancy

Definition

Preexisting hypertension or hypertension diagnosed before 20 weeks not attributed to trophoblastic diseases. Common causes include essential hypertension, renal diseases, connective tissue disorders—systemic lupus erythematosus (SLE), and endocrine cause—pheochromocytoma.

SCREENING AND PREVENTION OF PREECLAMPSIA

First Trimester Screening for Preeclampsia (Table 8)

Performance of screening for PE at 11-13.6 weeks of gestation by the Fetal Medicine Foundation (FMF) algorithm using a combination of maternal factors, mean arterial pressure (MAP), uterine artery pulsatility index (UTPI), PlGF, and serum pregnancy-associated plasma protein A (PAPP-A) is by far superior to the methods recommended by the National Institute for Health and Care Excellence (NICE) and the American College of Obstetricians and Gynecologists (ACOG). The algorithm was originally developed from a study of 58,884 singleton pregnancies at 11–13 weeks of gestation and further validated by study of 35,948 cases.[1] Detection rate for preterm PE and term PE of 75% and 43% false-positive rate (FPR) 10% MAP is calculated from SBP and DBP readings.

TABLE 8: ACOG 2020 recommendations.

Level of risk	Risk factors	Recommendations
High There is 8% or more risk of PE	History of preeclampsia, especially when accompanied by an adverse outcome: • Multifetal gestation • Chronic hypertension • Type 1 or 2 diabetes • Renal disease • Autoimmune disease (i.e., SLE and APLA syndrome) • Nulliparity	Recommend low-dose aspirin (LDA) if the patient has one or more of these high-risk factors
Moderate	• Obesity (body mass index >30) • Family history of preeclampsia (mother or sister) • Sociodemographic characteristics (African American race and low socioeconomic status) • Age 35 years or older • Personal history factors (e.g., low-birth-weight or small for gestational age, previous adverse pregnancy outcome, and >10-year pregnancy interval)	Consider LDA if the patient has more than one of these moderate risk factors
Low		Do not recommend LDA

(ACOG: American College of Obstetricians and Gynecologists; ALPA: antiphospholipid antibody; PE: preeclampsia; SLE: systemic lupus erythematosus)

The measured SBP and DBP will be automatically converted to MAP by the risk calculator.

$$MAP = DBP + (SBP - DBP)/3$$

MAP should be measured as part of the risk assessment for PE and it should be measured by validated automated and semiautomated devices.

Uterine artery pulsatility index is done at 11–13 weeks [crown–rump length (CRL) 42–84 mm]. The values are fed on to FMF software—risk score >1/100 is high risk and needs to be given 150 mg of aspirin at bed time till 36 weeks of gestation. If UTPI and PlGF—not possible—use maternal risk and MAP. Website for risk calculation of risk is as follows https://fetalmedicine.org/research/assess/PE.

Ophthalmic artery Doppler velocimetry has been used to predict the development of PE. Similar to Doppler studies of uterine arteries alone, ophthalmic artery Doppler velocimetry likely has little clinical utility as a standalone predictive test for either early or late on set PE.

Other preventive strategies include education about the signs and symptoms of PE and follow-up high-risk women with more frequent office visits. Loosing prepregnancy weight not exceeding recommendations for gestational weight gain (by National Academy of Medicine), reduce the chances of multiple gestation (if IVF) calcium 1 g/day and use of antioxidants.

MANAGEMENT OF PREECLAMPSIA WITH SEVERE FEATURES OR ECLAMPSIA[2]

Basic principles include:
- *Control of hypertension:* Severe hypertension—≥160/110 mm Hg, moderate—150–159/100–109 mm Hg, and mild—140–150/90–100 mm Hg.
- *Severe:* Antihypertensives always recommended because it is believed to reduce risk of maternal stroke. Intravenous (IV) labetalol is the drug of choice.

- *Mild-to-moderate:* Prudent approach is better which also considers the patient's comorbidities and symptoms (e.g., headache, visual disturbances, etc.). The benefits and potential risks of treatment are less clear. Aggressive lowering or medication themselves inhibit fetal growth and fetus is exposed to harmful effects of drugs.
- *Prevent or control seizure:* Magnesium sulfate is the drug of choice. Recommended regimen is 4 g IV in 100 mL, normal saline, 4 g intramuscular (IM); 2 g in each buttock as loading dose. Then 1 g/hour infusion till 24 hours after last convulsion or delivery whichever is later. Watch for magnesium toxicity by monitoring respiratory rate, urine output, and deep tendon reflexes. Magnesium sulfate overdose should be treated with 1 g calcium gluconate (10 mL of 10% solution).
- *Look for and treat renal, liver, and hematological involvement:* Needs magnesium sulfate prophylaxis and termination of pregnancy.
- *Identify fetal compromise:* Delivery is indicated if fetal condition is static or falling centiles. Doppler indices should be used to monitor fetus and decision for delivery to be taken based on fetal and maternal status.
- *Achieve meticulous fluid balance:* Risk of pulmonary edema due to reduced colloid osmotic pressure as a result of hypoalbuminemia, increased capillary permeability, and increased hydrostatic pressure. Fluid is not tolerated due to depleted plasma volume in PE. There is also risk of acute kidney injury. Total fluids should be restricted to 80 mL/hour, at least till postpartum diuresis occurs. An indwelling catheter should be inserted to monitor urine output, which should at least be 25 mL/hour.
- *Delivery:* It is the definitive treatment in patients with eclampsia or PE with severe features. Corticosteroids should be administered to improve lung maturity. Mode of delivery depends on fetal and maternal condition. Cesarean delivery indicated if there is severely growth restricted fetus, early preterm fetus (<34 weeks or 1,500 g), fetus in distress (BPP <5, AFI <5, AEDF in Doppler), presence of CPD, malpresentation or position and poor Bishop score. In practice, wherever neonatal intensive care unit (NICU) facilities are available with good survival rates for very-low-birth-weight babies the trend is toward cesarean.
- *Postpartum period:* Monitor BP closely. If features of severe PE present continue antihypertensive till BP normalizes. Magnesium sulfate needed if impending symptoms or eclampsia in postpartum period. Review patient after 2 weeks. Yearly BP, lipids, fasting blood sugar (FBS), and body mass index (BMI).

CONCLUSIONS

Diagnosis and timely management of hypertensive disorders of pregnancy is essential to prevent maternal and perinatal morbidity and mortality. Screening for preeclampsia should be followed routinely at 11–13.6 weeks.

REFERENCES

1. O'Gorman N, Wright D, Poon LC, Rolnik DL, Syngelaki A, de Alvarado M, et al. Multicenter screening for pre-eclampsia by maternal factors and biomarkers at 11-13 weeks' gestation: comparison with NICE guidelines and ACOG recommendations. Ultrasound Obstet Gynecol. 2017;49(6):756-60.
2. Landon M, Galan H, Jauniaux E, Driscoll D, Berghella V, Grobman W, et al. Gabbe's Obstetrics: Normal and Problem Pregnancies, 8th edition. Amsterdam, Netherlands: Elsevier; 2020.

Chapter 3

Diabetes in Pregnancy

Pawan Preet Mann Gill

■ INTRODUCTION

Diabetes mellitus (DM) is a rapidly increasing globally prevalent public health problem with rising prevalence among all age groups. The International Diabetes Federation (IDF) 2019 estimates that diabetes affects about 463 million people globally which is projected to increase to 642 million people by 2040.[1] In 2019, the global prevalence of hyperglycemia in pregnancy (HIP) in the age group 20–49 years was estimated to be 20.4 million or 15.8% of live births.[1] They had some form of HIP of which 83.6% were due to gestational diabetes mellitus (GDM).[1] GDM is defined as any degree of glucose intolerance with onset or first recognition during pregnancy.[1]

In India, GDM is detected in around 4 million pregnancies every year. The incidence of HIP (GDM and pre-GDM) parallels the prevalence of prediabetes, overweight, obesity, and type 2 diabetes in a given population. The increasing prevalence of DM is usually attributed to:
- The aging population structures
- Urbanization
- Obesity epidemic
- Physical inactivity
- Intrauterine exposure (gestational programming) is emerging as a potential risk factor.

Gestational programming is a process whereby stimuli (hyperglycemia) or stresses that occur at critical or sensitive periods of fetal development permanently change structure, physiology, and metabolism which predispose individuals to disease in adult life.

■ MATERNAL FETAL METABOLISM IN NORMAL PREGNANCY

In the pregnant woman, food intake initiates a complex series of hormonal actions due to the rise in blood glucose leading to secretion of pancreatic insulin, glucagon, somatomedins, and adrenal catecholamines. These adjustments aim at providing an ample, but not excessive, supply of glucose to the mother and fetus. Compared with nonpregnant counterparts, they have a higher tendency to develop hypoglycemia between meals and during sleep. This happens because the fetus continues to draw glucose across the placenta from the maternal blood stream even during periods of fasting.

Placental steroid and peptide hormones (estrogens, progesterone, and chorionic somatomammotropin) levels rise linearly throughout the second and third trimesters. This leads to increasing tissue insulin resistance, and by the third trimester, 24-hour mean insulin levels are 50% higher than the nonpregnant levels.

■ MATERNAL-FETAL METABOLISM IN DIABETES

If the maternal pancreatic insulin response to the increasing insulin resistance imparted by pregnancy hormones is inadequate, maternal and then fetal hyperglycemia results. This typically manifests as recurrent postprandial hyperglycemia episodes which lead to the accelerated growth exhibited by the fetus.

Maternal and fetal hyperglycemia leads to episodic fetal hyperinsulinemia which in turn promotes excess nutrients storage resulting in macrosomia. The energy expenditure associated with the conversion of excess glucose into fat causes depletion in fetal oxygen levels.

These episodes of fetal hypoxia provoke surges in adrenal catecholamines which further leads to hypertension, cardiac remodeling and hypertrophy, stimulation of erythropoietin, red cell hyperplasia, and increased hematocrit. High hematocrit values in the neonate lead to vascular sludging, poor circulation [postulated to be the cause of Intrauterine fetal demise (IUFD)], and postnatal hyperbilirubinemia.

CONSEQUENCES OF GESTATIONAL DIABETES MELLITUS

Maternal risks of GDM include polyhydramnios, preeclampsia, prolonged labor, obstructed labor, cesarean section, uterine atony, postpartum hemorrhage, and infection, which are the leading global causes of maternal morbidity and mortality. Progression of diabetic retinopathy and nephropathy can occur in pre-GDM patients. They are also at higher risk to develop cardiovascular diseases later in life. Fetal risks are enumerated in **Table 1**.

TABLE 1: Fetal risks related to diabetes.

Congenital abnormalities	*Neonatal complications*

• Cardiovascular:
  – TGA
  – Double outlet right ventricle
  – VSD
  – Truncus arteriosus
  – Tricuspid atresia
  – PDA
• Nervous system:
  – Neural tube defects (anencephaly, meningocele, and encephalocele)
  – Caudal regression syndrome
  – Holoprosencephaly
• Genitourinary system:
  – Renal agenesis
  – Hydronephrosis
  – Ureteral duplication
  – Cystic kidneys
• Gastrointestinal:
  – Duodenal atresia
  – Anorectal atresia
  – Small left colon syndrome
• Musculoskeletal system:
  – Arthrogryposis
  – Hypoplastic femur
	• Prematurity (spontaneous or iatrogenic)
	• Macrosomic/LGA infants
	• Birth complications and injuries:
	  – Perinatal hypoxia
	  – Respiratory distress
	• Metabolic complications:
	  – Hypoglycemia
	  – Hypocalcemia
	  – Hypomagnesemia
	  – Cardiomyopathy
	• Hematological complications:
	  – Polycythemia
	  – Low iron stores
	• Hyperbilirubinemia
	• Renal vein thrombosis
	• Adrenal hemorrhage

(LGA: large for gestational age; PDA: patent ductus arteriosus; TGA: transposition of the great arteries; VSD: ventricular septal defect)

SCREENING AND DIAGNOSIS

Despite the five international workshops devoted to GDM since 1979 there is considerable controversy surrounding identification of GDM. Both the screening and diagnostic criteria vary among countries and commonly between obstetric and diabetes organizations in a single country **(Table 2)**.

Indian Recommendations for Screening and Diagnosis

Universal Screening

In the yesteryears, it was aimed to recommend diagnostic cutoff values corelating to the future risk of T2 DM in the mother with less attention paid pregnancy outcomes,

TABLE 2: Current guidelines for screening and diagnosis for GDM.

Guideline, year	Range	No. of steps	OGTT criteria	OGTT timing	Risk factors list	Screening in early pregnancy
IADPSG, 2010	Global	One	FPG ≥92 mg/dL 1 hour ≥180 mg/dL and/or 2 hours ≥153 mg/dL Glucose load-75 g	24–28 weeks	Yes	FPG ≥92 mg/dL
WHO, 2013	Global	One	IADPSG	Any time	No	Same criteria apply at all times
FIGO, 2015	Global	One	IADPSG	24–28 weeks Or Any other time	Yes	Not applicable due to lack of clear evidence
NICE, 2015	UK	One	FPG ≥100 mg/dL Or 2-hour PG ≥140 mg/dL	24–28 weeks	Yes	75 g 2 hours OGTT in history of previous GDM asap after booking
ACOG, 2018	US	Two	1. Carpenter and Coustan (CC) 95-180-155-140 mg/dL (3 hours 100 g OGTT) 2. National Diabetes Data Group 104-190-165-144 mg/dL (4 hours 100 g OGTT) 2 or more values in both criteria	24–28 weeks	Yes	BMI >25 kg/m^2 (23 for Asian Americans) ≥1 additional risk factors
ADA, 2018	US	One/two	IADPSG/CC	24–28 weeks	Yes	OGTT for high risk women at first antenatal visit and classified as T1/T2 DM

(ACOG: American College of Obstetricians and Gynecologists; ADA: American Diabetes Association; BMI: body mass index; DM: diabetes mellitus; FIGO: International Federation of Gynecology and Obstetrics; FPG: fasting plasma glucose; GDM: gestational diabetes mellitus; IADPSG: International Association of the Diabetes and Pregnancy Study Group; NICE: National Institute for Health and Clinical Excellence; OGTT: oral glucose tolerance test; PG: postload glucose; WHO: World Health Organization) particularly among women with "mild gestational hyperglycemia". Studies in the last decade have shown significant association between adverse pregnancy outcomes and levels of maternal glucose considered within the nondiabetic range.

Therefore, universal and early testing in population with high prevalence of T2 DM is now recommended. Indian women have 11-fold increased risk of developing glucose intolerance during pregnancy compared to Caucasian women.[2] Among ethnic groups in South Asian countries, Indian women have the highest frequency of GDM.[3] Hence, the current recommendation is that all pregnant women should be screened for GDM even if they have no symptoms.[4]

Diabetes in Pregnancy Study Group India (DIPSI), a prospective study performed in India established that GDM can be diagnosed if 2-hour PG ≥140 mg/dL with 75 g oral glucose administered to pregnant women in the fasting or nonfasting state, irrespective of the last meal timing.[5] Rationale for this diagnostic test is that even after a meal, a normal glucose tolerant woman should be able to maintain euglycemia despite glucose challenge, due to brisk and adequate insulin response. Whereas a woman with GDM who has impaired insulin secretion, her glycemic level increases with a meal and with glucose challenge the glycemic excursion exaggerates further.

This "single test procedure" has been approved by the Ministry of Health, Government of India,[6] WHO,[7] IDF,[8] and International Federation of Gynecologists and Obstetricians society (FIGO).[9] The National Institute of Clinical Excellence (NICE) guidelines also recommend 2-hour PG >140 mg/dL as diagnostic criteria for GDM based on the study performed in multiethnic population of UK.[10]

TABLE 3: The screening timing.

Screening	Weeks of pregnancy
First	Ideally 12–16 weeks Or First antenatal visit
Second	24–28 weeks
Third	32–34 weeks

Protocol for Investigation (Table 3)

The first testing should be done during the first trimester as almost one-third of GDM women are detected during this period[11] or first antenatal contact, as early as possible in pregnancy. The chances are a few of them may have prediabetes. The second testing should be done during 24–28 weeks of pregnancy, if the first test is negative. It is important to ensure second test as many pregnant women develop glucose intolerance during this 24–28 weeks window. If it could not be done during this time, then it can be done any time later in pregnancy. There should be at least 4 weeks gap between any two tests. The test is to be conducted for all pregnant women if even if they come late in pregnancy for antenatal care (ANC) at the time of first contact. If she presents beyond 28 weeks of pregnancy, only one test is to be done at the first point of contact.

Type 1 Diabetes

The disease is typically diagnosed, in childhood or adolescence during an episode of hyperglycemia, ketosis, and dehydration. It is rare to be diagnosed during pregnancy. Patients diagnosed during pregnancy most often present with unexpected coma.

Type 2 Diabetes

According to the American Diabetes Association (ADA) the presence of any one of

the following criteria supports the diagnosis of DM:[12]
- Hemoglobin A1C (HbA1C) of 6.5% or greater
- Fasting plasma glucose (FPG) of 126 mg/dL or greater
- 2-hour PG level of 200 mg/dL or greater during a 75 g oral glucose tolerance test (OGTT)
- A random blood sugar RBS level of 200 mg/dL or greater in a patient suffering the classic symptoms of hyperglycemia or hyperglycemic crisis.

■ PREDIABETES

Women with prediabetes identified before pregnancy are at extremely high risk for developing GDM during pregnancy. As such they should receive early first trimester diabetic screening.

■ POST-DIAGNOSTIC TESTING

Once the diagnosis of diabetes is established in a pregnant woman, it is important to keep testing for glycemic control and diabetic complications for the rest of the pregnancy.

First Trimester Laboratory Studies
- HbA1C
- *Kidney function test* (KFT)—blood urea, serum creatinine, and urine albumin-creatinine ratio (ACR)
- Thyroid-stimulating hormone TSH and free thyroxine (FT4)
- Regular monitoring of blood sugar levels.

Second Trimester Laboratory Studies
- Urine ACR in women with elevated value in first trimester
- HbA1C
- Regular monitoring of blood sugar levels

Ultrasonography
- First trimester—dating and viability scan
- Second trimester—anomaly scan at 18–20 weeks and a fetal echocardiogram (22–24 weeks) if the maternal glycohemoglobin level value was elevated in the first trimester.
- Third trimester—growth scan to assess fetal size every 4–6 weeks starting from 26 weeks, in women with pre-GDM. Perform a growth ultrasonogram for fetal size at least once at 36–37 weeks for women with GDM.

Other Investigations

If maternal diabetes is longstanding or associated with known microvascular disease, obtain a baseline electrocardiogram (ECG), 2-D echo and fundus examination.

■ PREPREGNANCY MANAGEMENT FOR PREEXISTING DIABETES

Diabetic patients who wish to conceive should focus on good preconceptional control, because birth defects occur as early as 3–6 weeks after conception. Therapeutic goals are best achieved through a team approach. An effective diabetes management program should also include a thorough assessment of cardiovascular, renal, and ophthalmologic status. Frequent and regular monitoring of both preprandial and postprandial capillary glucose levels should be done with the following target glucose levels:[13]
- FPG 90–99 mg/dL

And
- 1 hour postprandial glucose (PPG) <140 mg/dL

Or
- 2-hour PPG <120–127 mg/dL.

The insulin regimen should aim at a smooth glucose profile throughout the day with no episodes of hypoglycemia between meals or at night. Initiate the regimen early enough so that the HbA1C level is lowered into the reference range for at least 3 months before conception.

Patients should take 1.0 mg of folic acid daily for at least 3 months before conception to minimize the risk of neural tube defects in the fetus. Counsel the nonpregnant women to avoid pregnancy until their HbA1C is <6.5%.

Dietary Therapy

The mainstay of dietary therapy is to avoid large meals and foods with a high content of simple carbohydrates. A total of six feedings per day is advised with three major meals and three snacks to limit the glucose load at each meal. The diet should include foods with complex carbohydrates and cellulose such as whole grain breads and legumes.

Carbohydrates should account for no >50% of the diet, with proteins and fats equally accounting for the remainder.[14,15] However, moderate restriction of carbohydrates to 35-40% has been shown to decrease maternal glucose levels and improve maternal and fetal outcomes.[16]

According to a randomized, placebo controlled study of pregnant women with GDM, supplemental calcium and vitamin D at 24-28 weeks gestation may have beneficial effects on metabolic profile [FPG, insulin, low-density lipoprotein (LDL), and high-density lipoprotein (HDL) levels].[17,18]

Insulin Therapy

Patients with pre-GDM require regular modification of their prepregnancy regimen to meet the changing metabolic demands of pregnancy. In patients with GDM, early intervention with insulin or an oral agent is the key to achieving a good outcome when diet therapy fails to provide adequate glycemic control.

The goal of insulin therapy during pregnancy is to achieve glucose profiles similar to those of nondiabetic pregnant women within a relatively narrow range (70-120 mg/dL).

Insulin lispro, aspart, regular, and neutral protamine Hagedorn (NPH) are well studied in pregnancy and regarded as safe and effective. Insulin glargine is less well studied and, given its long pharmacological effect, may exacerbate periods of maternal hypoglycemia.[19] Insulin detemir is safe and comparable to NPH insulin in pregnancy.[20]

The American College of Obstetricians and Gynecologists (ACOG) recommends starting with lispro insulin 4-8 units subcutaneously initially before meals. If >10 units of regular insulin is needed before the noon meal, add 8-12 units of NPH insulin before breakfast. When >10% of fasting glucose levels exceed 95 mg/dL, initiate 6-8 units NPH insulin at bedtime. Titrate doses as needed according to blood glucose levels.[19]

Insulin Pump

In a selected group of patients, use of an insulin pump may improve glycemic control while enhancing patient convenience. These devices can be programmed to infuse varying basal and bolus levels of insulin, which change smoothly even while the patient sleeps or is otherwise preoccupied.

Oral Therapy

The efficacy and safety of insulin have made it the standard for treatment of diabetes during pregnancy. Nevertheless, the oral agents glyburide and metformin are gaining popularity. Trials have shown these agents to be effective and no evidence of harm to the fetus has been found, although the potential for long-term adverse effects remains a concern.[21]

Glyburide: Glyburide is a second-generation sulfonylurea that is minimally transported across the human placenta. A 2,000 randomized trial comparing glyburide to insulin in 404 pregnancies found no difference between the groups in mean maternal blood glucose levels, the percentage of infants who were large for gestational age (LGA), birth weights, or neonatal complications. Only 4% of patients in the glyburide study arm required addition of insulin to achieve glucose control.22 Several prospective and retrospective studies involving >775 pregnancies have concluded that glyburide is as safe and effective as insulin.

Glyburide should not be used in the first trimester, because its effects, if any, on the embryo are unknown. Glyburide has been shown to be safe in breastfeeding, with no transfer into human milk. However, Indian recommendations do not yet include glyburide.

Metformin: Metformin is a biguanide, which functions mainly by decreasing hepatic glucose output. Metformin crosses the placenta, and umbilical cord levels have been shown to be even higher than maternal levels.[23]

Metformin is associated with a lower risk of neonatal hypoglycemia and less maternal weight gain than insulin. However, in 2015 systematic review, metformin was found to have a slight increase in the risk of prematurity. Furthermore, nearly half of patients with GDM who were initially treated with metformin in randomized trial needed insulin in order to achieve acceptable glucose control.

As metformin reduces insulin resistance and has the potential to lower the risk of ensuing GDM in polycystic ovary syndrome (PCOS) mothers, its role appears truly encouraging. According to the ADA, when used to treat PCOS and induce ovulation, metformin needs not be continued once pregnancy has been confirmed but Indian perspective is in contrast. Most of the obstetricians in India prefer to continue metformin even after the women conceives based on their experience. According to the results from the PregMet-2 study, the drug appeared to reduce the risk for late miscarriage and preterm birth in PCOS, although the percentage of women taking metformin who developed GDM (25%) approximately matched that of women taking a placebo (24%).[24]

Metformin may be used as a safe and effective oral hypoglycemic agent in GDM, especially in low-resource settings where cost, storage, and compliance are logistic issues.[25] Metformin therapy was not associated with increased adverse pregnancy outcomes in women with type 2 diabetes mellitus (T2DM) as compared with standard insulin therapy.[26] Metformin is recommended by the national guidelines in the "Diagnosis and Management of GDM" (Ministry of Health, Government of India).[27]

MANAGEMENT OF GDM— INDIAN GUIDELINES

Guiding Principles

- All pregnant women who test positive for GDM for the first time should be started on medical nutrition therapy (MNT) and physical exercise for 2 weeks. The woman should walk or exercise for 30 minutes daily or perform household work.
- If 2 hours postprandial plasma glucose remains >120 mg/dL with MNT and lifestyle changes, metformin or insulin therapy is recommended.

TABLE 4: Energy requirement of gestational diabetes mellitus (GDM) women.

Level of activity	Energy requirement + Pregnancy requirements	Total energy requirement (kcal/day)
Sedentary work	1,900 + 350	2,250
Moderate work	2,230 + 350	2,580
Heavy work	2,850 + 350	3,200

Medical Nutrition Therapy

An easy method **(Table 4)** for the dietary guidelines for primary healthcare providers.

Pharmacological Therapy

- Metformin or insulin therapy is the accepted medical management of pregnant women with GDM not controlled on MNT. Insulin is the first drug of choice.
- Insulin can be started anytime during pregnancy for GDM if MNT fails.
- If pregnant woman is not willing for insulin, metformin can be recommended provided gestational age is >12 weeks.[25] The starting dose of metformin is 500 mg twice daily orally up to a maximum of 2 g per day. If the woman's blood sugar is not controlled with the maximum dose of metformin and MNT, there is no other option but to advise insulin. Metformin is recommended by the national guidelines in the "Diagnosis and Management of GDM" (by Ministry of Health, Government of India).[27]

Monitoring Glycemic Control when on MNT or Metformin

- After satisfactory glycemic control is achieved, monitoring at least once a month may be performed.
- Every 2 weeks between 24th and 28th week of gestation.
- Every week after 28th week till delivery.

Insulin Therapy

- The recommended starting dose of insulin in GDM is 0.1 unit per kg of body weight per day.
- Repeat FPG and 2-hour PPPG every third day. Add 2U prebreakfast if PPPG is raised and add 2U predinner if FPG is raised after every third day testing.
- Continue testing and increasing insulin dose till desired levels of FPG <90 and 2-hour PPPG <120 mg/dL are achieved.
- Rarely a GDM woman requires >20 units of insulin per day. If she requires multiple doses of insulin, it is prudent to involve a physician.
- Pre-GDM (T1DM and T2DM) may require premeal regular insulin and bedtime basal insulin or premixed insulin twice a day is an option.
- Insulin analogs are safer during pregnancy.

Target Glycemic Control

The success of prevention of T2DM entirely depends on aiming for target glycemic level, that is, maternal glucose should be maintained similar to nondiabetic pregnant women. It has been documented that occurrence of macrosomia has a continuous relationship to the 2-hour PG above 120 mg/dL [adjusted odds ratio 3.02 (95% CI 1.30–7.0), p <0.05][28,29] and to FPG which becomes significant above 90 mg/dL [adjusted odds ratio 2.08 (95% CI 1.24–3.48), p = 0.005].[30,31] FBG <90 mg/dL prevents macrosomia as well as other adverse outcomes, such as preeclampsia and contrary to belief, neonatal hypoglycemia does not occur in women with GDM.[32] The ACOG also recommends fasting ≤90 mg/dL and 2-hour PG ≤120 mg/dL similar to DIPSI target.[33-34]

PRENATAL OBSTETRIC MANAGEMENT

Periodic Fetal Biophysical Testing

The goals of management of diabetic pregnancies in third trimester pregnancies are to prevent stillbirth and asphyxia and to minimize maternal and fetal morbidity associated with delivery. Fetal growth needs to be monitored to select the proper timing and route of delivery. This is accomplished by frequent testing for fetal well-being and serial ultrasonographic examinations to follow fetal size.

Various fetal biophysical tests are available to the clinician to ensure that the fetus is well oxygenated **(Table 5)**. If applied properly, most of these tests along with fetal umbilical Doppler ultrasonographic studies can be used with confidence to provide assurance of fetal well-being while awaiting fetal maturity.

In patients with poor glycemic control, intrauterine growth restriction (IUGR), or significant hypertension, formal biophysical testing should start as early as 28 weeks. In patients who are at lower risk, formal fetal testing can begin at 34 weeks.

Fetal Growth Assessment

Despite problems with accuracy, ultrasonogram-based estimation of fetal size has become the standard of care. Estimate fetal size once or twice at least 3 weeks apart in order to establish a trend. Time the last examination to be at 36–37 weeks of gestation or as close to the planned delivery date as possible.

TIMING AND ROUTE OF DELIVERY

Benefits of delaying the delivery to as near as possible to the estimated date of delivery (EDD) are better cervical maturity, improved chances of spontaneous labor, and vaginal delivery. However, the risks of advancing fetal macrosomia, birth injury, and in utero demise increase as the due date approaches.

If the fetus is not macrosomic and the results of biophysical testing are reassuring, the obstetrician can await spontaneous labor. In patients with GDM and superb glycemic control, continued fetal testing and expectant management can be considered until 41 weeks gestation (ACOG). In the fetuses with an abdominal circumference significantly larger than the head circumference or an estimated fetal weight above

TABLE 5: Biophysical tests of fetal well-being for diabetic pregnancy.

Test	Frequency	Reassuring result	Comment
Fetal movement counting	Every night from 28 weeks	10 movements in <60 minutes	Performed in all patients
Nonstress test (NST)	Twice weekly	Two fetal heart rate (FHR) accelerations in 20 minutes	• 28–34 weeks onward in insulin-dependent diabetes • 36 weeks onward in diet controlled gestational diabetes mellitus (GDM)
Contraction stress test	Weekly	No FHR deceleration in response to three contractions in 10 minutes	Same as for NST
Ultrasonographic biophysical profile	Weekly	Score of 8 in 30 minutes	• 3 movements = 2 • 1 flexion = 2 • 30 seconds breathing = 2 • 2 cm amniotic fluid = 2

4,000 g, consider induction. After 40 or more weeks, the benefits of continued conservative management are likely to be outweighed by the danger of fetal compromise.

An optimal time for delivery of most diabetic pregnancies is typically on or after the 39th week. Deliver a patient with diabetes before 39 weeks of gestation without documented fetal lung maturity only for compelling maternal or fetal indications. The ACOG recommends offering cesarean delivery to diabetic patients if the fetal weight is estimated to be 4,500 g or more.

INTRAPARTUM GLYCEMIC MANAGEMENT

Intrapartum maternal hyperglycemia is directly proportional to neonatal hyperinsulinemia and subsequent hypoglycemia. Avoiding hyperglycemia during labor can therefore dramatically reduce the incidence of neonatal hypoglycemia. A combined insulin and glucose infusion should be used during labor to maintain maternal blood sugars in a narrow range (70–110 mg/dL). Typical infusion rates are 5% dextrose in ringer lactate solution at 100 mL/h and regular insulin at 0.5–1.0 U/h. Blood sugar levels are monitored hourly in these patients.

For patients with diet controlled GDM or mild T2DM, avoiding dextrose in intravenous fluids normally suffices to maintain excellent blood glucose control without any need for insulin-glucose infusion.

MANAGEMENT OF THE NEONATE

The most critical metabolic problem that affects infants of diabetic mothers is hypoglycemia. Unmonitored and uncorrected hypoglycemia can lead to neonatal seizures, brain damage, and death. Thus, current recommendations specify frequent blood glucose checks and early oral feeding when possible ideally from the breast, with infusion of intravenous glucose if oral measures prove insufficient. Most neonatologist maintain strict monitoring of the glucose levels of newborn infants of diabetic mothers for at least 4–6 hours and frequently 24 hours, often necessitating neonatal intensive care unit (NICU) admission. Evidence indicates that breastfed infants have a much lower risk of developing diabetes than those exposed to cow's milk proteins. Studies of breastfeeding women with diabetes indicate that lactation even for a short duration also has a beneficial effect on overall maternal glucose and lipid metabolism. This may reduce the future diabetes risk after GDM.

POSTPARTUM CARE

All GDM women should be tested for glucose intolerance 6 weeks after delivery. In the postpartum period, the single test procedure which was followed in the antepartum period can be followed. If 75 g OGTT is done, she should be diagnosed to have impaired fasting glucose (IFG) if FPG is >100 mg/dL and diagnosed as impaired glucose tolerance (IGT) if 2 hour PPG is >140 mg/dL.

If GDM woman is on insulin, she may not require insulin immediately after the delivery and in the postpartum period. GDM woman who was on metformin may be advised to continue if her PPG is high ($\geq$140 mg/dL). Metformin can be continued during breastfeeding. It is well documented that women with GDM have a very high risk of developing T2DM and cardiovascular disease postpartum. This risk can be reduced by promoting weight loss and through breastfeeding. Women with diabetes have delayed milk production and lower rates of breastfeeding. Therefore lactation support should be offered to these patients.

PREVENTION OF GESTATIONAL DIABETES MELLITUS

Prevention of GDM is an attractive concept but no progress has been made despite attempts in small studies. Because body fat and diet contribute to the risk of GDM, patients who lose weight before pregnancy and follow an appropriate diet may lower their risk of GDM. However, the hormone levels in pregnancy impose such a high degree of insulin resistance, that in very susceptible individuals, even marked weight loss and attention to diet are not likely to be successful. Additionally, a large study by Stafne et al. found that a 12-week standard exercise program during the second half of pregnancy had no benefit in preventing GDM in healthy women with normal body mass index (BMI).[35]

CONCLUSION

There is a continuously and exponentially increasing incidence of diabetes in pregnancy. Universal screening, strict management and patient education can go a long way in reducing the obstetric impact as well as overall burden of diabetes in the society and it's next generation.

REFERENCES

1. International Diabetes Federation. IDF Diabetes Atlas, 9th edition. Brussels, Belgium: International Diabetes Federation; 2019.
2. Dornhost A, Paterson CM, Nicholls JS, Wadsworth J, Chiu DC, Eikeles RS, et al. High prevalence of gestational diabetes in Women from ethnic minority groups. Diabet Med. 1992;9(9):820-5.
3. Beischer NA, Oats JN, Henry OA, Sheedy MT, Walstab JE. Incidence and severity of gestational diabetes mellitus according to country of birth in women living in Australia. Diabetes. 1991;40 Suppl 2:35-8.
4. Fiore K. United States Preventive Service Task force (USPSTF) Backs Universal Diabetes Screening. 2014.
5. Anjalakshi C, Balaji V, Balaji MS, Ashlatha S, Sunganthi S, Arthi T, et al. A single test procedure to diagnose gestational diabetes mellitus. Acta Diabetol. 2009;46:51-4.
6. Mishra S, Bhadoria AS, Kishor S, Kumar R. Gestational diabetes mellitus 2018 guidelines: An update. J Family Med Prim Care. 2018;7:1169-72.
7. Colagiuri S, Falavigna M, Agarwal MM, Boulvain M, Coetzee E, Hod M, et al. Strategies for Implementing the WHO Diagnostic Criteria and Classification of Hyperglycaemia First Detected in Pregnancy. Diabetes Res Clin Pract. 2014;103(3):364-72.
8. Hod M, Kapur A, Sacks DA, Hadar E, Agarwal M, Di Renzo GC, et al. The International Federation Of Gynecology and Obstetrics (FIGO) Initiative on Gestational Diabetes Mellitus: a Pragmatic Guide for Diagnosis, Management, and Care. Int J Gynaecol Obstet. 2015;131 Suppl 3:S173-211.
9. Sadikot S, Purandare CN, Cho NH, Hod M. FIGO-IDF joint statement and declaration on hyperglycemia in pregnancy. Diabetes Res Clin Pract. 2018;145:1-4.
10. National Institute for Health and Care Excellence: Guidelines. London: National Institute for Health and Care Excellence (NICE); 2015.
11. Singh N, Madhu M, Vanamail P, Malik N, Kumar S. Efficacy of Metformin in improving glycemic control & perinatal out come in gestational diabetes mellitus: a non-randomized study. Indian J Med Res. 2017;145:623-8.
12. American Diabetes Association Professional Practice Committee. 2. Classification and Diagnosis of Diabetes: Standards of Medical Care in Diabetes-2022. Diabetes Care. 2022;45(Suppl 1):S17-38.
13. Metzger BE, Gabbe SG, Persson B, Buchanan TA, Catalano PA, Damm P, et al. International association of diabetes and pregnancy study group recommendations on the diagnosis and classification of hyperglycemia in pregnancy. Diabetes Care. 2010;33(3):676-82.
14. American Diabetes Association. Standards of Medical Care in Diabetes—2010. Diabetes Care. 2010;33 Suppl 1:S11-61.

15. American Diabetes Association. Standards of Medical Care in Diabetes—2013. Diabetes Care. 2013:36 Suppl 1:S11-66.
16. Meltzer SJ, Snyder J, Penrod JR, Morin L. Gestational diabetes mellitus diagnosis and screening: a prospective randomised controlled trial comparing costs of one-step and two-step methods. BJOG. 2010;117(4):407-15.
17. Henderson D. (2014). GDM: Vitamin D, Calcium Combo Improves Metabolic Profile. [online] Available from https://www.medscape.com/viewarticle/827316. [Last accessed April, 2023].
18. Asemi Z, Karamali M, Esmaillzadeh A. Effects of Calcium-Vitamin D co-supplementation on glycemic control, inflammation and oxidative stress in gestational diabetes: a randomised placebo-controlled trial. Diabetologia. 2014;57(9):1798-806.
19. Cheung NW. The management of gestational diabetes. Vasc Health Risk Mang. 2009;5(1):153-64.
20. Mathiesen ER, Hod M, Ivanisevic M, Duran Garcia S, Brondsted L, Jovanovic L, et al. Maternal Efficacy and Safety Outcomes in a Randomised Controlled Trial Comparing Insulin Detemir with NPH Insulin in 310 pregnant women with Type 1 Diabetes. Diabetes Care. 2012;35:2012-7.
21. Moore LE, Clokey D, Rappaport VJ, Curent LB. Metformin compared with glyburide in gestational diabetes: a randomised controlled trial. Obstet Gynecol. 2010;115(1):55-9.
22. Langer O, Conway DL, Berkus MD, Xenakis EM, Gonzales O. A comparison of glyburide and insulin in women with gestational diabetes mellitus. N Engl J Med. 2000;343(16):1134-8.
23. Vanky E, Zahlsen K, Spigset O, Carlsen M. Placental passage of metformin in women with polycystic ovary syndrome. Fertil Steril. 2005;83(5):1575-8.
24. Tucker ME. Metformin May Prevent Pregnancy Complications in PCOS. [online] Available from https://www.medscape.com/viewarticle/894316. [Last accessed April, 2023].
25. Veeraswamy S, Divakar H, Gupte S, Datta M, Kapur A, Vijayam B. Need for testing glucose tolerance in the early weeks of pregnancy. Indian J Endocrinol Metab. 2016;20(1):43-6.
26. Lin SF, Chang SH, Kuo CF, Lin WT, Chiou MJ, Huang YT. Association of pregnancy outcomes in women with type 2 diabetes treated with metformin versus insulin when becoming pregnant. BMC Pregnancy Childbirth. 2020;20(1):512.
27. Seshiah V, Balaji V, Balaji MS, Paneerselvam A, Kapur A. Pregnancy and diabetes scenario around the world: India. Int J Gynaecol Obstet. 2009;104 Suppl 1:S35-8.
28. Balaji V, Balaji MS, Seshiah V, Mukundan S, Datta M. Maternal glycemia and neonate's birth weight in Asian Indian women. Diabetes Res Clin Pract. 2006;73(2):223-4.
29. de Sereday MS, Damiano MM, Gonzalez CD, Bennett PH. Diagnostic criteria for gestational diabetes in relation to pregnancy outcome. J Diabetes Complications. 2003;17:115-9.
30. Seshiah V, Balaji V, Balaji MS, Panneerselvam A. Abnormal Fasting Plasma Glucose during pregnancy. Diabetes Care. 2008;31(12):e92.
31. Lapolla A, Dalfra MG, Bonomo M, Castiglioni MT, Cianni GD, Masin M, et al. Can plasma glucose and HbA1C predict fetal growth in mothers with different glucose tolerance levels? Diabetes Res Clin Pract. 2007;77:465-70.
32. Prutsky GJ, Domecq JP, Wang Z, Carranza Leon BG, Elraiyah T, Nabhan M, et al. Glucose targets in pregnant women with diabetes: a systematic review and meta-analysis. J Clin Endocrinol Metab. 2013;98:4319-24.
33. Herandez TL, Friedman JE, Van Pelt RE, Barbour LA. Patterns of glycemia in normal pregnancy: Should the current therapeutic targets be challenged? Diabetes Care. 2011;34(7):1660-8.
34. Gunderson EP, Hedderson MM, Chiang V, Crites Y, Walton D, Azevedo RA, et al. Lactation intensity and postpartum maternal glucose tolerance and insulin resistance in women with recent GDM: The SWIFT cohort. Diabetes Care. 2012;35(1):50-6.
35. Stafne SN, Salvesen K, Romundstad PR, et al. Regular exercise during pregnancy to prevent gestational diabetes: A randomized controlled trial. Obstet Gynecol. 2012;119(1):29-36.

Chapter 4

Obesity in Pregnancy

Revati Nitin Rane

■ INTRODUCTION

Obesity has become a global epidemic and obesity in pregnancy has become the most common medical problem in pregnancy. It is a unique challenge in obstetrics, considering its prevalence and potential adverse effects on mother and fetus during pregnancy and in later life.

MATERNAL OBESITY: WORLDWIDE STATISTICS

2016 world report on noncommunicable diseases indicated that prevalence of obesity in women has increased from 6.4 to 14.9%.[1] European region's current prevalence of maternal obesity ranges from 7 to 25%.[2] First trimester maternal obesity is more than doubled from 7.6 % to 15.6%.[3]

OBESITY GENERAL CONSIDERATION

Most often used system to classify obesity is *body mass index (BMI)* or *Quetelet index* which is calculated as weight in kilograms divided by square of the height in meters (kg/m^2).

■ CLASSIFICATION

According to the National Institute of Health (2000) the classification of obesity is as mentioned in **Table 1**.

TABLE 1: Classification of obesity.

Category	BMI (kg/m^2)
Normal	18.5–24.9
Overweight	25–29.9
Obesity	≥30
• Class 1	30–34.9
• Class 2	35–39.9
• Class 3 (morbid obesity)	≥40
Super morbid obesity	≥50

(BMI: body mass index)

■ DEFINITION

Obesity in pregnancy is defined as BMI of 30 kg/m^2 or more using prepregnancy height and weight or if not available the measured parameters at first antenatal visit.[4-7]

MANAGEMENT OF OBESITY IN PREGNANCY

Prepregnancy

In prepregnancy period, preexistent obesity complications affect the course and outcome of pregnancy. They should be looked for, corrected, and optimization for pregnancy should be advocated.

Preexisting Complications Caused by Obesity before Pregnancy

- Menstrual irregularities, anovulation, subfertility and infertility,[8] decreased

pregnancy, and live birth rates when undergoing assisted reproductive technology (ART)[9]
- Cardiac dysfunction, proteinuria, and nonalcoholic fatty liver[10]
- Obstructive sleep apnea (OSA)[11]
- Pregestational diabetes and hypertension
- Oral contraceptive failure is more likely.

Nonalcoholic fatty liver disease (NAFLD) deserves a special mention as it is associated with high obstetric complications.[12] High proportion of low-density lipoprotein (LDL) level is the hallmark of NAFLD so LDL levels require special attention.

Preconceptional Counseling

- Obese woman should be counseled regarding the implications of BMI on fertility and pregnancy outcomes and expected maternal and fetal complications.
- Patients should be counseled regarding nutrition and exercise program should be discussed.[4-7,13-15]
- Society of obstetricians and gynaecologists of Canada (SOGC) specifically recommends encouraging prepregnancy BMI of <25–30 kg/m^2.[7]
- Planning and necessity of bariatric surgery should be discussed with experts as from observational studies fertility rates improve and obstetric complication rates decline in women after bariatric surgery compared to morbidly obese controls.[16]
- Post-bariatric surgery, nutritionist should be consulted for vitamin supplementation before and during pregnancy[4,6,17] as risk of preterm labor and small for gestational age newborn increases postsurgery.[18-20]
- The American College of Obstetricians and Gynecologists (ACOG) recommends screening for OSA[11] before planning pregnancy or at first antenatal visit.

Antepartum Complications and Antenatal Care

Excess gestational weight gain (GWG) is associated with adverse obstetric outcomes.[21] Women with prepregnancy overweight and obesity are more likely to gain excess weight during pregnancy.[22,23] Recommendation for GWG in pregnancy by the American College of Obstetrics and Gynecology (ACOG) are as per the recommendations given by United States of Medicine in 2009 and they are as follows and are independant of age, parity, smoking, race, and ethnicity. GWG targets should be calculated and discussed with women early in pregnancy.

The United States of America Institute of Medicine recommendation 2009 for total weight gain during pregnancy as per prepregnancy BMI is given in **Table 2**.

Antenatal Complications

The complications associated with obesity in antenatal period in mothers and fetus are as described in **Table 3**.

TABLE 2: Target weight gain.

Prepregnancy BMI	BMI	Total weight gain (kg)
Underweight	<18.5	12.7–18
Normal weight	18.5–24.9	11.3–15.9
Overweight	25–29.9	6.8–11.3
Obesity class 1, 2 and 3	>30	5–9

(BMI: body mass index)

TABLE 3: Antenatal complications.

Maternal	Fetal
Miscarriage[24]	• Congenital defects[30,31] • Increased risk of neural tube defects[32-34]
Gestational diabetes mellitus[25]	Increased risk for trisomy 21[35]
Pregnancy-induced hypertension[26,27]	large for gestational age macrosomia[36]
Preeclampsia[28]	Small for gestational age
Thromboembolism[29]	Premature birth[37]

Keeping in mind the mentioned complications recommendation for antenatal care for obese patient as per international guidelines are:
- The Royal College of Obstetricians and Gynecologists (RCOG) and the Royal Australian and New Zealand College of Obstetricians and Gynecologists (RANZCOG) recommend high dose preconceptional folic acid supplementation of 5 mg/day for women preconceptionally and throughout antenatal period.[32-34] The ACOG differs and recommends the routine dose.
- The RCOG recommends vitamin D supplementation of 10 µg daily.[38]
- The RANZCOG recommends 150 µg iodine daily.[6,39]
- The RANZCOG recommends vaccination against H1N1 during pregnancy considering high risk in pregnancy with obesity.[40]
- The ACOG recommends early screening of glucose intolerance and repeat screening at 24–28 weeks.[4,32]
- The RCOG recommends surveillance of preeclampsia.
- *Low dose aspirin:* As per the RCOG recommendations, obesity qualifies as moderate risk factor for preeclampsia as per the National Institute for Health and Care Excellence (NICE) guidelines on hypertensive disorder.[41] So when especially paired with other risk factors such as age >40 years, multiple gestations, family history, and low-dose aspirin of 75 mg at 12 weeks of gestation should be started[41] along with adequate calcium intake.[42,43]
- The ACOG recommends low-molecular-weight heparin (LMWH) prophylaxis in antenatal period on an individually assessed basis.[4,44,45]
- After contraindications to exercise have been ruled out, an eventual goal of moderate intensity exercise for 20–30 minutes per day for 3–5 days a week can be advised.[46]
- Considering the risk of still birth and concurrent diabetes and hypertension, close fetal monitoring is indicated in later gestation.
- *Obesity and preterm labor:* It is often iatrogenic and is related to medical comorbidities but there is also an increase in spontaneous extreme preterm labor (<28 weeks of gestation)[47] which is attributed to increased inflammatory markers and increased risk of bacterial infections and chorioamnionitis. Screening and treatment of bacterial vaginosis should be done.

Intrapartum Complications and its Management

Obesity causes complications in mother in labor and to be born baby which are summarized in **Table 4**.

TABLE 4: Intrapartum complications and its management.

Maternal	Fetal
Preterm labor[48]	Prematurity
Postdated pregnancy	Stillbirth[49,50]
Labor inductions twice likely (Denison 2008)	Neonatal trauma due to macrosomia and shoulder dystocia[51,52]
Failure of inductions (Wolfe 2011)	Meconium aspirations and ventilatory support (Marshall 2014 Smid 2016)
More chances of cesarean delivery (26 vs. 40%)[53-56]	Low Apgar at 5 and 10 minutes[51]
Prolonged labor[56,57]	
Low success of VBAC[47-50]	

(VBAC: vaginal birth after cesarean)

Timing of Delivery

Decision of time of delivery in obese pregnant patient is multifactorial. With 10 units increase in prepregnancy BMI there is associated twofold increase in stillbirth risk.[51] Few studies suggest that induction at 38–39 weeks is associated with low neonatal complications.[52]

The ACOG and RCOG both concluded that in absence of other obstetric or medical indication, obesity alone is not an indication for induction and spontaneous labor should be encouraged.[5,53]

Surgical Management

Cesarean delivery is riskier and more difficult in women with obesity. The availability of specialized surgical instruments, weight capacity equipment such as operating theater (OT) tables and wheel chairs, etc., should be available in the setup.

Choice of Incision

Both transverse and vertical incisions are associated with advantages and disadvantages as compared in **Table 5**, so the choice of incision should be decided on a case-to-case basis.

Difficulties and Safety during Anesthesia

Both regional and general anesthesia impose various risks and difficulties. Regional anesthesia may have difficulties because of adiposity and changed landmarks and lead to multiple failed attempts, so sometimes ultrasound guided techniques might help.

General anesthesia is associated with difficult intubations in up to 33% of obese pregnant patients,[54] attributed to increased breast mass, chest diameter, and exaggerated airway edema.

Postpartum Management

Vigilant postpartum management is important in obese patients for good fetomaternal outcome. Complications should be kept in mind are discussed here.

Postpartum Complications

Obesity not only causes antenatal and intranatal problems but it also imposes significant postpartum complications as described in **Table 6**.

TABLE 5: Incision during cesarean section.

	Transverse	Vertical
Wound strength	More	Less
Postoperative pain	Less	More
Postoperative respiratory status	Better, with less pain	Less, associated with more pain
Retraction during surgery	Difficult	Easy
Baby delivery	Difficult	Easy
Wound infection rate	Similar	Similar

TABLE 6: Postpartum complications.

Maternal	Fetal
Postpartum hemorrhage[55-57]	Risk of hypoglycemia
Difficulty in initiation and sustaining breastfeeding[58]	Increased admission rates in NICU[59]
Peripartum heart failure (Cunningham 1986, 2012)	Increased neonatal deaths[38,60-63]
Increased Wound infections[55]	
Postpartum depression[55]	
Venous thromboembolism[29]	
Maternal deaths	

(NICU: neonatal intensive care unit)

The risk of postpartum hemorrhage (PPH) is almost doubled in obese pregnant patients after both vaginal and operative delivery.[64] Risk of PPH is increased with fetal weight, Asian ethnicity, and attributed to traumatic and atonic causes. There are no universal guidelines on prophylaxis for venous thromboembolism (VTE).

The ACOG recommends pneumatic mechanical compression prior to following cesarean section.[65] Consideration of LMWH should be done in very high-risk cases on an individual basis.[65]

The RCOG recommends 1 week of LMWH for all women with BMI >40 kg/m² regardless of mode of delivery. For BMI >30 kg/m² with one or more clinical risk factor as per clinical Green-Top guidelines; 7 days postdelivery LMWH prophylaxis is given.

Breastfeeding

Breastfeeding is helpful for mothers with obesity for various reasons as it is associated with decrease in:
- Cardiovascular risk[66]
- Type 2 diabetes mellitus (DM)[67,68]
- Visceral obesity in later life.[69,70]

Difficulties in breastfeeding in these patients are caused by insufficient breast glandular tissue and psychosocial factors.

■ LONG-TERM COMPLICATIONS

Obesity has been associated with various complications which are seen in later part of mother and fetus as stated in **Table 7**.

Obesity and children's neurodevelopmental outcome are studied in various studies and meta-analysis concluded that high fat diet and prepregnancy obesity and excess weight gain during pregnancy is related to the adverse neurodevelopmental outcome of the baby.[72]

Neurodevelopmental problems such as attention deficit and hyperactivity disorder (ADHD), autism spectrum disorder (ASD), emotional and behavioral problems are 17% higher in overweight and 51% higher in obese pregnant patients.[73]

TABLE 7: Long-term complications.

Maternal	Fetal
Postpartum weight retention	Childhood obesity
Type 2 diabetes mellitus (DM)	Premature metabolic Syndrome[71]
Long-term vascular dysfunction[26,27]	Premature deaths from cardiovascular diseases[3]
	Adverse neurodevelopmental outcomes

There is an increase in worldwide prevalence of overweight and obesity. Current estimate suggests that by 2038 about 38% of world's population is expected to be obese.

Obesity is a systemic and psychosocial condition that has massive effect on maternal morbidity and mortality as well as outcomes of generations to come.

Healthcare professionals should help patients openly discuss about this sensitive issue and provide safe medical care with appropriate resources, customized equipment's and definitive protocols with multidisciplinary approach.

■ REFERENCES

1. NCD Risk Factor Collaboration (NCD-RisC). Trends in adult body-mass index in 200 countries from 1975 to 2014: a pooled analysis of 1698 population-based measurement studies with 19.2 million participants. Lancet. 2016;387:1377-96.
2. Devlieger R, Benhalima K, Damm P, Van Assche A, Mathieu C, Mahmood T, et al. Maternal obesity in Europe: where do we stand and how to move forward?: a scientific paper commissioned by the European Board and College of Obstetrics and Gynaecology (EBCOG). Eur J Obstet Gynecol Reprod Biol. 2016;201:203-8.

3. Heslehurst N, Rankin J, Wilkinson JR, Summerbell CD. A nationally representative study of maternal obesity in England, UK: trends in incidence and demographic inequalities in 619 323 births, 1989-2007. Int J Obes (Lond). 2010;34:420-8.
4. American College of Obstetricians and Gynecologist. Obesity in Pregnancy: ACOG Practice Bulletin No 495. Obstet Gynecol. 2015;126:e112-26.
5. Centre for Maternal and Child Enquiries, Royal College of Obstetricians and Gynaecologist. CMACE/RCOG Joint Guideline: Management of Women with Obesity in Pregnancy. Wales: CMACE/RCOG; 2010.
6. The Royal Australian and New Zealand College of Obstetricians and Gynaecologists. (2013). Management of Obesity in Pregnancy. [online] Available from https://ranzcog.edu.au/wp-content/uploads/2022/05/Management-of-Obesity-in-Pregnancy.pdf. [Last accessed April, 2023].
7. Davies GA, Maxwell C, McLeod L, Gagnon R, Basso M, Bos H, et al. SOGC Clinical Practice Guidelines: Obesity in pregnancy. No. 239, February 2010. Int J Gynaecol Obstet. 2010;110(2):167-73.
8. Talmor A, Dunphy B. Female obesity and infertility. Best Pract Res Clin Obstet Gynaecol. 2015;29:498-506.
9. Rittenberg V, Seshadri S, Sunkara SK, Sobaleva S, Oteng-Ntim E, El-Toukhy T. Effect of body mass index on IVF treatment outcome: an updated systematic review and meta-analysis. Reprod Biomed Online. 2011;23(4):421-39.
10. Catalano PM. Management of obesity in pregnancy. Obstet Gynecol 2007;109:419-33.
11. Pien GW, Pack AI, Jackson N, Maislin G, Macones GA, Schwab RJ. Risk factors for sleep disordered breathing in pregnancy. Thorax. 2014;69:371-7.
12. Hagström H, Höijer J, Ludvigsson JF, Bottai M, Ekbom A, Hultcrantz R, et al. Adverse outcome of pregnancy in women with nonalcoholic fatty liver disease. Liver Int. 2016;36:268-74.
13. Piirainen T, Isolauri E, Lagstrom H, Laitinen K. Impact of dietary counselling on nutrient intake during pregnancy: a prospective cohort study. Br J Nutr. 2006;96:1095-104.
14. Dodd JM, Turnbull D, McPhee AJ, Deussen AR, Grivell RM, Yelland LN, et al. Antenatal lifestyle advice for women who are overweight or obese: LIMIT randomised trial. BMJ. 2014;348:g1285.
15. Davies GAL, Wolfe LA, Mottola MF, MacKinnon C. Exercise in pregnancy and the postpartum period. J Obstet Gynaecol Can. 2003;25:516-22.
16. Komoniarek MA, Jungheim ES, Hoeger KM, Rogers AM, Kahan S, Kim JJ, et al. American Society for Metabolic and Bariatric surgery position statement on the impact of obesity and obesity treatment on fertility and fertility therapy. Endorsed by American College of Obstetricians and Gynecologist and the Obesity Society. Surg Obes Relat Dis. 2017;13(5):750-7.
17. Weissman A, Hagay Z, Schacter M, Dreazen E. Severe maternal and fetal electrolyte imbalance in pregnancy after gastric surgery for morbid obesity: a case report. J Rep Med. 1995;40(11):813-6.
18. Yi XY, Li QF, Zhang J, Wang ZH. A meta-analysis of maternal and fetal outcomes of pregnancy after bariatric surgery. Int J Gynaecol Obstet. 2015;130(1):3-9.
19. Kjaer MM, Lauenborg J, Breum BM, Nilas L. The risk of adverse pregnancy outcome after bariatric surgery: a nationwide register-based matched cohort study. Am J Obstet Gynecol. 2013;208(6):464.e1-5.
20. Roos N, Neovius M, Cnattingius S, Lagerros YT, Sääf M, Granath F, et al. Perinatal outcomes after bariatric surgery: nationwide population based matched cohort study. BMJ. 2013;347:f6460.
21. Ferraro ZM, Contador F, Tawfiq A, Adamo KB, Gaudet L. Gestational weight gain and medical outcomes of pregnancy. Obstet Med. 2015;8(3):133-7.
22. Weisman CS, Hillemeier MM, Downs DS, Chuang CH, Dyer AM. Preconception predictors of weight gain during pregnancy: prospective findings from the Central Pennsylvania Women's Health Study. Womens Health Issues. 2010;20(2):126-32.

23. Ferraro ZM, Barrowman N, Prud'homme D, Walker M, Wen SW, Rodger M, et al. Excessive gestational weight gain predicts large for gestational age neonates independent of maternal body mass index. J Matern Fetal Neonatal Med. 2012;25(5):538-42.
24. Boots C, Stephenson MD. Does obesity increase the risk of miscarriage in spontaneous conception: a systematic review. Semin Reprod Med. 2011;29:507-13.
25. Kennelly MA, McAuliffe FM. Prediction and prevention of Gestational Diabetes: an update of recent literature. Eur J Obstet Gynecol Reprod Biol. 2016;202:92-8.
26. Chandrasekaran S, Levine LD, Durnwald CP, Elovitz MA, Srinivas SK. Excessive weight gain and hypertensive disorders of pregnancy in the obese patient. J Matern Fetal Neonatal Med. 2015;28:964-8.
27. Bohrer J, Ehrenthal DB. Other adverse pregnancy outcomes and future chronic disease. Semin Perinatol. 2015;39:259-63.
28. O'Brien TE, Ray JG, Chan WS. Maternal body mass index and the risk of preeclampsia: a systematic overview. Epidemiology. 2003; 14:368-74.
29. Robinson HE, O'Connell CM, Joseph KS, McLeod NL. Maternal outcomes in pregnancies complicated by obesity. Obstet Gynecol. 2005;106:1357-64.
30. Watkins ML, Rasmussen SA, Honein MA, Botto LD, Moore CA. Maternal obesity and risk for birth defects. Pediatrics. 2003;111 (5 Pt 2):1152-8.
31. Stothard KJ, Tennant PW, Bell R, Rankin J. Maternal overweight and obesity and the risk of congenital anomalies: a systematic review and meta-analysis. JAMA. 2009;301: 636-50.
32. National Institute of Health and Clinical Excellence. (2010). Weight management before, during and after pregnancy. [online] Available from https://www.nice.org.uk/guidance/ph27/resources/weight-management-before-during-and-after-pregnancy-pdf-1996242046405. [Last accessed April, 2023].
33. Rasmussen SA, Chu SY, Kim SY, Schmid CH, Lau J. Maternal obesity and risk of neural tube defects: a metaanalysis. Am J Obstet Gynecol. 2008;198(6):611-9.
34. Mojtabai R. Body mass index and serum folate in childbearing age women. Eur J Epidemiol. 2004;19(11):1029-36.
35. Hildebrand E, Kallen B, Josefsson A, Gottvall T, Blomberg M. Maternal obesity and risk of Down syndrome in the offspring. Prenat Diagn. 2014;34(4):310-5.
36. Oken E. Maternal and child obesity: the causal link. Obstet Gynecol Clin North Am. 2009;36:361-77.
37. Faucher MA, Barger MK. Gestational weight gain in obese women by class of obesity and select maternal/newborn outcomes: asystematic review. Women Birth. 2015;28:e70-9.
38. O'Reilly JR, Reynolds RM. The risk of maternal obesity to the long-term health of the offspring. Clin Endocrinol (Oxf). 2013;78:9-16.
39. National Health and Medical Research Council. Iodine supplementation for Pregnant and Breastfeeding Women: Public statement. Canberra: National Health and Medical Research Council; 2010.
40. The Royal Australian and New Zealand College of Obstetricians and Gynaecologists. Influenza Vaccination during Pregnancy (C-Obs 45). Melbourne, Australia: The Royal Australian and New Zealand College of Obstetricians and Gynaecologists; 2011.
41. National Institute for Health and Clinical Excellence. Hypertensive disorders during pregnancy. London: National Institute for Health and Clinical Excellence; 2010.
42. Magee LA, Pels A, Helewa M, Rey E, von Dadelszen P; Canadian Hypertensive Disorders of Pregnancy Working Group. Diagnosis, evaluation, and management of the hypertensive disorders of pregnancy: executive summary. J Obstet Gynaecol Can. 2014;36(7):575-6.
43. Cantu JA, Jauk VR, Owen J, Biggio JR, Abramovici AR, Edwards RK, et al. Is low-dose aspirin therapy to prevent preeclampsia more efficacious in non-obese women or when initiated early in pregnancy? J Matern Fetal Neonatal Med. 2015;28(10):1128-32.

44. Duhl AJ, Paidas MJ, Ural SH, Branch W, Casele H, Cox-Gill J, et al. Antithrombotic therapy and pregnancy: consensus report and recommendations for prevention and treatment of venous thromboembolism and adverse pregnancy outcomes. Am J Obstet Gynecol. 2007;197:457e1-21.
45. Practice Bulletin No. 123: Thromboembolism in pregnancy. Obstet Gynecol. 2011;118:718-29.
46. American College of Obstetricians and Gynecologists. ACOG committee opinion no. 650: physical activity and exercise during pregnancy and the postpartum period. Obstet Gynecol. 2015;126(6):e135-142.
47. Cnattingius S, Villamor E, Johansson S, Edstedt Bonamy AK, Persson M, Wikström AK, et al. Maternal obesity and risk of preterm delivery. JAMA. 2013;309(22): 2362-70.
48. McDonald SD, Han Z, Mulla S, Beyene J, Knowledge Synthesis G. Overweight and obesity in mothers and risk of preterm birth and low birth weight infants: systematic review and meta-analyses. BMJ. 2010;341: c3428.
49. Chu SY, Kim SY, Lau J, Schmid CH, Dietz PM, Callaghan WM, et al. Maternal obesity and risk of stillbirth: a metaanalysis. Am J Obstet Gynecol. 2007;197:223-8.
50. Kumari AS. Pregnancy outcome in women with morbid obesity. Int J Gynaecol Obstet. 2001;73:101-7.
51. Lutsiv O, Mah J, Beyene J, McDonald SD. The effects of morbid obesity on maternal and neonatal health outcomes: a systematic review and metaanalyses. Obes Rev. 2015; 16:531-46.
52. Gottlieb AG, Galan HL. Shoulder dystocia: an update. Obstet Gynecol Clin North Am. 2007;34:501-31.
53. Dietz PM, Callaghan WM, Morrow B, Cogswell ME. Population-based assessment of the risk of primary cesarean delivery due to excess pre-pregnancy weight among nulliparous women delivering term infants. Matern Child Health J. 2005;9:237-44.
54. Hibbard JU, Gilbert S, Landon MB, Hauth JC, Leveno KJ, Spong CY, et al. Trial of labor or repeat cesarean delivery in women with morbid obesity and previous cesarean delivery. Obstet Gynecol. 2006;108:125-33.
55. Chu SY, Kim SY, Schmid CH, Dietz PM, Callaghan WM, Lau J, et al. Maternal obesity and risk of cesarean delivery: a meta-analysis. Obes Rev. 2007;8:385-94.
56. Yu CK, Teoh TG, Robinson S. Obesity in pregnancy. BJOG. 2006;113(10):1117-25.
57. Nuthalapaty FS, Rouse DJ, Owen J. The association of maternal weight with cesarean risk, labor duration, and cervical dilation rate during labor induction. Obstet Gynecol. 2004;103:452-6.
58. Durnwald CP, Ehrenberg HM, Mercer BM. The impact of maternal obesity and weight gain on vaginal birth after cesarean section success. Am J Obstet Gynecol. 2004;191: 954-7.
59. Juhasz G, Gyamfi C, Gyamfi P, Tocce K, Stone JL. Effect of body mass index and excessive weight gain on success of vaginal birth after Cesarean delivery. Obstet Gynecol. 2005;106:741-6.
60. Chauhan SP, Magann EF, Carroll CS, Barrilleaux PS, Scardo JA, Martin JN Jr. Mode of delivery for the morbidly obese with prior cesarean delivery: vaginal versus repeat cesarean section. Am J Obstet Gynecol. 2001;185:349-54.
61. Goodall PT, Ahn JT, Chapa JB, Hibbard JU. Obesity as a risk factor for failed trial of labor in patients with previous cesarean delivery. Am J Obstet Gynecol. 2005;192(5):1423-6.
62. Carmichael SL, Blumenfeld YJ, Mayo J, Wei E, Gould JB, Stevenson DK, et al. Prepregnancy obesity and risks of stillbirth. PLoS One. 2015;10(10):e0138549.
63. Lee VR, Niu B, Anjali K, Little S, Nicholson J, Caughey AB. Optimal timing of delivery in obese women: a decision analysis. Obstet Gynecol. 2014;123(S1):152S-3S.
64. ACOG Practice Bulletin No. 107: Induction of labor. Obstet Gynecol. 2009;114:386-97.
65. Tan T, Sia AT. Anesthesia considerations in the obese gravida. Semin Perinatol. 2011;35(6):350-5.
66. Sebire NJ, Jolly M, Harris JP, Wadsworth J, Joffe M, Beard RW, et al. Maternal obesity and pregnancy outcome: a study of 287,213

pregnancies in London. Int J Obes Relat Metab Disord. 2001;25(8):1175-82.
67. Usha Kiran TS, Hemmadi S, Bethel J, Evans J. Outcome of pregnancy in a woman with an increased body mass index. BJOG. 2005;112(6):768-72.
68. Blomberg M. Maternal obesity and risk of postpartum hemorrhage. Obstet Gynecol. 2011;118:561-8.
69. Lepe M, Bacardi Gascon M, Castaneda-Gonzalez LM, Perez Morales ME, Jimenez Cruz A. Effect of maternal obesity on lactation: systematic review. Nutr Hosp. 2011;26:1266-9.
70. Hancke K, Gundelach T, Hay B, Sander S, Reister F, Weiss JM. Pre-pregnancy obesity compromises obstetric and neonatal outcomes. J Perinat Med. 2015;43:141-6.
71. Leddy MA, Power ML, Schulkin J. The impact of maternal obesity on maternal and fetal health. Rev Obstet Gynaecol. 2008;1: 170-8.
72. Catalano PM, Ehrenberg HM. The short- and long-term implications of maternal obesity on the mother and her offspring. Br J Obstet Gynaecol. 2006;113:1126-33.
73. Scott-Pillai R, Spence D, Cardwell C, Hunter A, Holmes V. The impact of body mass index on maternal and neonatal outcomes: a retrospective study in a UK obstetric population, 2004–2011. BJOG. 2013;120:932-9.

Chapter 5

Thyroid Disorders in Pregnancy

Neema Acharya, Sourya Acharya, Samarth Shukla

■ INTRODUCTION

Changes in Thyroid Function During Pregnancy

Pregnancy is associated with adaptive changes in most of the systems during pregnancy one of them being thyroid function.[1] There is physiologic increase in size of thyroid gland almost up to 30% attributed to hypotrophy and fluid collection.

During pregnancy maternal total or bound thyroid hormone levels increase along with levels of thyroid-binding globulin. The level of thyroid-stimulating hormone (TSH) decreases in early pregnancy which is mainly due to high levels of human chorionic gonadotropin (hCG) found in first trimester. Also there is increase in serum free thyroxine (T4) levels which leads to suppression of thyroid releasing hormone reducing TSH levels. After the first trimester, TSH levels return to nonpregnant level and increase at the end of pregnancy due to release of placental deiodinase.

While interpreting thyroid tests these physiologic changes should be taken into consideration.[2]

Population-based trimester-specific reference ranges for serum TSH should be defined for every population after studying levels of only thyroid tests results of pregnant women with normal thyroid function.[3] Table 1 summarizes the reference points to be taken while concluding results of thyroid tests in pregnancy.

Fetal Brain Development

Almost 30% of T4 found in umbilical cord blood at birth comes from mother. Before the fetal thyroid starts its action, fetal brain growth is dependent of maternal T4 transferred through placenta. Neonates of women who are being treated with antithyroid medication should be screened for neonatal thyroid function.[4,5]

■ HYPERTHYROIDISM

Incidence of hyperthyroidism in pregnancy is reported as 0.2–0.7%. Out of these almost 95% are diagnosed as Graves' disease.

Table 2 summarizes the clinical features of hyperthyroidism. Most of the symptoms

TABLE 1: Consideration for adjusting reference points in pregnancy.[1]

Hormone	Lower reference point	Upper reference point	Trimester
Thyroid-stimulating hormone (TSH)	Lowered by 0.4 mU/L than normal	Lowered by 0.5 mU/L than normal	First trimester
Total T4	–	Increased by 50%	Second trimester
Total T3	–	Increased by 50%	Second trimester

TABLE 2: Symptoms of hyperthyroidism.		
Hyperthyroidism	Symptoms	Signs
	Nervousness, frequent stools, excessive sweating, heat intolerance, weight loss, insomnia, and palpitations	Tremors, tachycardia, goiter, and hypertension
Graves' disease		Ophthalmopathy dermopathy

and signs may delay diagnosis as these are also present physiologically during pregnancy. Laboratory tests should be done to confirm diagnosis. Uncontrolled maternal thyrotoxicosis is associated with pre-eclampsia, cardia failure, and thyroid storm.[6]

Fetal and Neonatal Effects

Uncontrolled hyperthyroidism is associated with medical complications in pregnancy. This leads to higher incidence of poor perinatal outcome related to first trimester abortions and preterm birth and rarely stillbirth. Persistent fetal tachycardia and fetal growth restriction warrant monitoring for fetal thyrotoxicosis. Thyroid-stimulating immunoglobulin and TSH binding inhibitory immunoglobulins found in mothers having Graves' disease get transmitted to fetus and affect the fetal thyroid.[7]

Subclinical Hyperthyroidism

The reported incidence is 0.8–1.7% during pregnancy. The laboratory findings show low serum TSH levels with normal free T4 levels. Presently evidence does not support treatment of subclinical hyperthyroidism. In addition, there are theoretical risks to the fetus because antithyroid medications cross the placenta and may adversely affect fetal thyroid function.[8]

Treatment of Overt Hyperthyroidism in Pregnancy

Either propylthiouracil or methimazole, both thioamides are used for treatment of pregnancy with overt hyperthyroidism. The choice of medication is dependent on gestational age at diagnosis, and type of thyrotoxicosis (predominantly T4 or T3).

Methimazole typically is category D drug in first trimester as it is known to cause multiple birth defects (aplasia cutis) and is best avoided in first trimester. In such cases propylthiouracil is preferred. Propylthiouracil preferentially decreases T4 to T3 conversion hence is used for treatment of T3-predominant thyrotoxicosis.

While switching the drug in preexisting disease a dose ratio of 20:1 propylthiouracil to methimazole is recommended. Propranolol should be added if there symptoms like palpitation anxiety. During pregnancy pregnancy total T3 level is found 1.5 times the non-pregnant normal level.

■ HYPOTHYROIDISM

Almost 2–10 per 1,000 pregnancies are affected by hypothyroidism. This entity is diagnosed when TSH level is above the upper reference point of normal and free T4 below the lower reference point.

Table 3 shows clinical features of thyroid deficiency. Hashimoto thyroiditis is found in iodine deficiency zones. Maternal and fetal production of T4 is dependent on adequate iodine intake. The recommended daily allowance of iodine is 220 μg during pregnancy while it is 290 μg during lactation.[9]

The evidence is inconclusive about supplementation of iodine routinely. In controlled, maternal hypothyroidism is

TABLE 3: Sign and symptoms of hypothyroidism.		
Hypothyroidism	Symptoms	Signs
	Fatigue, constipation, cold intolerance, muscle cramps, and weight gain	Edema, dry skin, hair loss, and a prolonged relaxation phase of deep tendon reflexes
Hashimoto thyroiditis		Goiter

associated with poor pregnancy outcomes in the form of abortions, accidental hemorrhage, preterm birth, and poor Apgar score of neonates. Multidisciplinary management of thyroid disease in pregnancy with adequate control of disease is shown to improve perinatal outcome.

Fetal and Neonatal Effects

Unlike hyperthyroidism the transmission of autoantibodies through placenta leading fetal affection is rare in maternal hypothyroidism. The occurrence of fetal hypothyroidism in the offspring of women with Hashimoto thyroiditis is noted to be approximately 1 in 180,000 neonates.

Subclinical Hypothyroidism

It is defined as serum TSH level higher than normal values whereas free T4 level is found normal. The incidence is estimated to be 2–5% in pregnancy. Current evidence does not support treatment of this entity during pregnancy.[10]

Treatment of Overt Hypothyroidism in Pregnancy

Hormone T4 therapy is started as levothyroxine at the dose of 1–2 µg/kg per day or 100 µg daily.

Patients who have undergone thyroidectomy or radiation treatment should be treated with replacement therapy and may require higher than normal dose to maintain normal function assessed through TSH levels. A goal of TSH level is to maintained between lower level up to 2.5 mU/L. Monitoring of TSH is done at 4–6 weeks of interval till normal for maintenance of goal. The T4 replacement dose is increased in one-third of hypothyroid pregnant women who were on preexistent treatment.

CLINICAL CONSIDERATIONS AND RECOMMENDATIONS

Screening for Thyroid Disorder during Pregnancy

Present evidence does not support screening for all pregnant women. Indications to test thyroid function during pregnancy are women with a personal or family history of thyroid disease, type 1 diabetes mellitus, or clinical suspicion of thyroid disease in the form of visible goiter or nodule in thyroid.

Laboratory Tests for Thyroid Disease during Pregnancy

- The first-line and most reliable screening test to assess thyroid status should be measurement of the TSH level.
- When the TSH level is abnormally high or low, free T4 level should be performed to determine if there is overt thyroid dysfunction.
- In cases of suspected hyperthyroidism, total T3 is preferred over free T3.
- The T3 and T4 levels should be maintained at upper limit while treating hyperthyroidism in pregnancy.

TABLE 4: Clinical features of thyroid storm.

Symptoms of thyroid storm	Signs of thyroid storm
Fever, palpitation, and breathlessness	1. Tachycardia 2. Dysrhythmia 3. Central nervous system affection cardiac failure 4. Pulmonary hypertension and cardiomyopathy

THYROID STORM AND THYROTOXIC HEART FAILURE IN PREGNANCY

This is a life-threatening disease.

As shown in **Table 4,** out of all clinical manifestations heart failure and pulmonary hypertension in pregnancy than the occurrence of thyroid storm in pregnancy. The reported incidence is 9% during pregnancy having uncontrolled hyperthyroidism. The obstetrics high-risk factors such as anemia, preeclampsia, and sepsis are the precipitating factors. Treatment is mainly done in intensive care area in multidisciplinary mode. Evidence suggests avoiding delivery in the presence of thyroid storm unless there is emergency obstetrics indication.

■ THYROID FUNCTION IN THE FETUS

Fetal screening for thyroid size by ultrasound or invasive cord blood sampling is not recommended by present guidelines. Umbilical cord blood sampling should be considered when there is high index of suspicion of fetal thyroid affection on ultrasound.

THYROID NODULE OR THYROID CANCER DURING PREGNANCY

Thyroid nodules are found in 1–2% of reproductive-aged women. Fortunately, 90–95% of solitary thyroid nodules are diagnosed as benign. Multidisciplinary approach should be followed for such a high risk pregnancy.

Majority of thyroid malignancies are well differentiated and have a course of slow progression. Thyroidectomy is treatment of choice if indicated in first and second trimester. Surgical treatment can be deferred to postpartum period if it is diagnosed in third trimester.

■ POSTPARTUM THYROIDITIS

Postpartum thyroiditis is defined as thyroid dysfunction within 12 months of delivery that can include clinical evidence of hyperthyroidism, hypothyroidism, or both. Approximately 5–10% of postpartum women during the first year postnatally show symptoms and signs of thyroid disease. The clinical scenario in immediate postpartum period is like thyrotoxicosis which later on after about 6–8 months ends into symptoms and signs of hypothyroidism.

In case of postpartum depression which lasts for long clinicians should consider evaluation of thyroid function. Most of the cases of thyroiditis resolve spontaneously and require temporarily antithyroid drugs.

These patients should be treated in multidisciplinary approach and kept under their observation and monitoring.

■ KEY POINTS

- Universal screening for thyroid disease in pregnancy is not recommended unless indications found on history and clinical examination.
- History of thyroid disease, multiple endocrine disease or evidence of clinical signs and/or suspicious signs of thyroid disease are indications for thyroid screening during pregnancy.
- In indicated cases, thyroid status in pregnancy should be assessed by measurement of the TSH level.

- The TSH level is maintained at lower end of normal limit and at 2.5 mU/L. Monitoring of TSH levels is done at 4–6 weeks interval.
- Overt hypothyroidism is treated to maintain the above said limit of TSH.
- Overt hyperthyroidism is treated to prevent adverse maternal and perinatal outcomes and drug of choice is as per the trimester of pregnancy taking into consideration risk of fetal anomalies.
- Hyperemesis gravidarum does not warrant thyroid function testing unless clinical signs are suspicious of same.

REFERENCES

1. Alexander EK, Pearce EN, Brent GA, Brown RS, Chen H, Dosiou C, et al. 2017 Guidelines of the American Thyroid Association for the Diagnosis and Management of Thyroid Disease During Pregnancy and the Postpartum. Thyroid. 2017;27(3): 315-89.
2. Carney LA, Quinlan JD, West JM. Thyroid disease in pregnancy. Am Fam Physician. 2014;89(4):273-8.
3. Tsakiridis I, Giouleka S, Kourtis A, Mamopoulos A, Athanasiadis A, Dagklis T. Thyroid Disease in Pregnancy: A Descriptive Review of Guidelines. Obstet Gynecol Surv. 2022;77(1):45-62.
4. Huget-Penner S, Feig DS. Maternal thyroid disease and its effects on the fetus and perinatal outcomes. Prenat Diagn. 2020;40(9):1077-84.
5. Wang Y, Sun XL, Wang CL, Zhang HY. Influence of screening and intervention of hyperthyroidism on pregnancy outcome. Eur Rev Med Pharmacol Sci. 2017;21(8):1932-7.
6. Kriplani A, Buckshee K, Bhargava VL, Takkar D, Ammini AC. Maternal and perinatal outcome in thyrotoxicosis complicating pregnancy. Eur J Obstet Gynecol Reprod Biol. 1994;54(3):159-63.
7. Turunen S, Vääräsmäki M, Lahesmaa-Korpinen AM, Leinonen MK, Gissler M, Männistö T, et al. Maternal hyperthyroidism and pregnancy outcomes: A population-based cohort study. Clin Endocrinol (Oxf). 2020;93(6):721-8.
8. López-Muñoz E, Mateos-Sánchez L, Mejía-Terrazas GE, Bedwell-Cordero SE. Hypothyroidism and isolated hypothyroxinemia in pregnancy, from physiology to the clinic. Taiwan J Obstet Gynecol. 2019;58(6): 757-63.
9. Dong AC, Morgan J, Kane M, Stagnaro-Green A, Stephenson MD. Subclinical hypothyroidism and thyroid autoimmunity in recurrent pregnancy loss: a systematic review and meta-analysis. Fertil Steril. 2020;113(3):587-600.e1.
10. Thyroid Disease in Pregnancy: ACOG Practice Bulletin, Number 223. Obstet Gynecol. 2020;135(6):e261-74.

6
Asthma in Pregnancy

Jyoti Jaiswal, Supriya Gupta

■ INTRODUCTION

Asthma is one of the common chronic medical conditions associated with pregnancy. It has affected 262 million people in 2019 and caused 455,000 deaths.[1] Asthma is defined as a chronic medical disorder of airways. Prevalence in pregnancy may range from 8 to 10% in developed countries to as high as 15–18% in developing countries.[2] This number, however, could be underestimated just as in nonpregnant women as many of them go unreported.

The World Health Organization (WHO) response for this health problem is that asthma is included in package of essential noncommunicable disease (PEN) for assessment, diagnosis, and management of chronic respiratory diseases (asthma and chronic obstructive pulmonary disease), especially in low resource countries.[1]

■ PATHOPHYSIOLOGY

Asthma is increased responsiveness of tracheobronchial tree, may have acute episode followed by a symptom-free interval. The course of asthma in pregnancy is related to the changes in the respiratory system during pregnancy **(Table 1)**.

Pregnancy is a state of physiological respiratory alkalosis, due to progesterone-mediated respiratory center stimulation. In this there is decreased arterial partial pressure of carbon dioxide, decreased bicarbonate, and increased pH.[3]

Along with anatomical and physiological changes, some immunological changes also occur in pregnancy from Th1-type cytokine production and toward Th2-type immune responses, which is mandatory for the fetus to survive. The Th2 upregulation and other immunity changes may lead to bronchial asthma exacerbation during pregnancy.[4]

There are four types of asthma severity as defined by the Centers for Disease Control and Prevention (CDC), i.e., intermittent, mild persistent, moderate persistent, and severe persistent.[5]

This classification is based on symptom, night time frequency, lung capacity, and inhaler use.
1. *Intermittent:* Symptoms 2 days or less a week and not interfere with regular activities. Forced expiratory volume (FEV) lung capacity test is usually 80% or more of normal values. Less than two times use of short-acting beta agonist (SABA).
2. *Mild persistent:* Symptoms will occur more often than twice a week but not every day. These symptoms tend to wake a person three or four times a month. Symptoms may have a minor impact on regular activities. The result of a FEV lung capacity test is often 80% or more of normal values. A person will need to use a SABA inhaler to control symptoms more often than twice a week but not daily.

Asthma in Pregnancy

TABLE 1: Physiological changes in the respiratory system.

1. Upper respiratory tract	Mucosal edema, hyperemia, and fragility upper airway	This begins from first trimester, peaks in late third trimester due to hyperestrogenic effect. 20% rhinosinusitis in pregnancy
2. Changes in thorax		
Diaphragm	4 cm pushed up	Increased uterine size elevates diaphragm
Chest diameter	Increased by 2 cm	Compensates for diaphragm elevation
Subcostal angle	Increased by 50%	
3. Changes in lung volume		
Minute ventilation	Increased 30–50%	
Tidal volume (TV)	Increased 40%	
Oxygen consumption	Increased 20%	
Functional residual capacity (FRC)	Decreased 20%	
Total lung capacity (TLC)	No change to decreased 5%	
Forced vital capacity (FVC)	No change	
Vital capacity (VC)	No change	
Forced expiratory volume in 1 second (FEV1)	No change	
Peak expiratory flow rate (PEFR)	No change	
Diffusing capacity of lungs for carbon monoxide (DLCO)	No change	
Respiratory rate (RR)	No change	

3. *Moderate persistent:* Symptoms will occur on a daily basis. Symptoms will wake a person more often than once a week but not every night. Symptoms will limit regular activities somewhat. The result of a FEV lung capacity test tends to be 60–80% of normal values. A person will need to use a SABA inhaler on a daily basis.
4. *Severe persistent:* Symptoms will arise throughout the day. A person will likely be woken by symptoms every night. Symptoms will significantly limit regular activities. The result of a forced vital capacity (FVC) lung function test tends to be <60% of normal values. A person will need to use a SABA inhaler to control symptoms several times a day.

■ COURSE DURING PREGNANCY

Asthma may progress, remain unchanged, or show improvement during pregnancy. Rule of one third in asthma: one-third worsening of their bronchial asthma during pregnancy, one-third without change in severity, and one-third their bronchial asthma shows improvement from the basal condition.

■ ASTHMA AND PREGNANCY

Relation of asthma and pregnancy is depicted in **Table 2**.

Diagnosis of Asthma in Pregnancy

Clinical features and various objective tests help in decision making. Symptoms include

TABLE 2: Relation of asthma and pregnancy.[6]	
Asthma on pregnancy	• Increased risk of preterm delivery • Increased risk of preeclampsia • Increased risk of hyperemesis gravidarum • Increased risk of vaginal bleeding • Increased risk of complicated labor • Increased risk of congenital malformation • Increased risk of asthma in offspring
Pregnancy on asthma	• Increased asthma-related hospitalizations than • Nonpregnant asthmatic cases • One-third worsening of their bronchial asthma during pregnancy • One-third, without change in severity • One-third, their bronchial asthma shows improvement from the basal condition
Risk factors for worsening of asthma during pregnancy	• Young age • Unmarried • Low socioeconomic condition • Poorly controlled/severe asthma prior to pregnancy • Gastroesophageal reflux disease

breathlessness, chest tightness, wheeze, shortness of breath, and cough. These symptoms have variability over time and intensity which worse at night or early in the morning, may or may not be triggered by allergen or viral infections.[6]

On physical examination may have wheeze on auscultation, with very severe cases present with silent chest as a result of severe reduction of airflow.

Variability in airflow can be confirmed by bronchodilator reversibility, bronchial provocation tests, and peak expiratory flow rate (PEFR) variability with airflow limitation.

Differential Diagnosis

The following should be considered:[3]
- Gastroesophageal reflux disease
- Hyperventilation syndrome
- Pulmonary embolism.

EVALUATION OF ASTHMA IN PREGNANCY

Clinical and Physical Examination

Diagnosis and severity of asthma in pregnancy should always be on the basis of clinical history and examination findings supported by spirometry as in case of nonpregnant females.

Objective Tests

Spirometry, lung volume measurement, and diffusing capacity of lungs for carbon monoxides (DLCO) testing are the primary pulmonary function tests (PFTs).[6]

- *Spirometry:* It is used for initial evaluation and diagnosis in a patient presenting with pulmonary symptoms. The initial evaluation of a patient with suspected reactive airway disease includes spirometry before and after bronchodilator therapy. Measurement of the forced expiratory volume in 1 second (FEV1) and FVC is included in spirometry. The ratio of FEV1/FVC is important in differentiating obstructive from restrictive airway disease (decreased vs. normal ratio, respectively). For follow-up outpatient visits, spirometry is preferable.
- *DLCO:* It assesses gas exchange within the lungs. Decreased DLCO is found with intrinsic lung disease, which is uncommon in pregnancy. The DLCO is essentially unchanged during pregnancy.[4]

- *PEFR:* It is an objective measure of airflow resistance and a surrogate measure of the FEV1. It can measure with small, inexpensive, and easy-to-use device. The normal PEFR for reproductive age women ranges from 380 to 500 L/min, which can be lower in the supine pregnant woman compared with those obtained while sitting or standing.
- *Pulse oximetry:* The oximetry system determines arterial oxygen saturation by measuring the absorption of selected wavelengths of light in pulsatile blood flow. Oxyhemoglobin absorbs much less red and slightly more infrared light than reduced hemoglobin. Oxygen saturation is the ratio of red to infrared absorption. Under ideal circumstances, most oximeters measure saturation to within 2% of arterial oxygen saturation.[7]
- Fractional exhaled nitric oxide (FeNO) and blood eosinophil counts are important tools for asthma assessment. FeNO is an indicator of airway inflammation. Adjusting treatment of asthma in pregnancy according to FeNO can reduce acute attacks and neonatal admission rate.[8]
- The methacholine challenge test is contraindicated during pregnancy as it may lead to acute bronchospasm.[3]

Patient Based Tools

Asthma Control Test (ACT): Apart from spirometry, ACT can be used in pregnancy which is 4 weeks recall symptom and daily functioning self-recalled patient-based questionnaire. It is a 22 item questionnaire with 5–25, with 25 indicating complete control. As a screening tool, the overall agreement between ACT and the specialist's rating ranged from 71 to 78% depending on the cut points used. Generally, if score is <20 it indicates uncontrolled asthma.[9]

MANAGEMENT OF ASTHMA DURING PREGNANCY

Goal of management is to provide optimal therapy for asthma control:
- No or minimal chronic symptoms, day or night
- Minimal or no exacerbations (exacerbations day or night, e.g., addition of oral corticosteroids, unscheduled outpatient visits, and admission to emergency department)
- No limitation of activity
- Maintenance of normal (near) pulmonary function
- Minimal use of short-acting beta-2 agonist inhaled
- Avoid maternal hypoxia to maintain adequate fetal oxygenation
- Minimal or no adverse effects of treatment provided
- Education and awareness regarding treatment and appropriate use of medications.

Management in Prenatal Period

Counseling, patient education, and adequate control are the key steps in prenatal period. It should be communicated to the patient that pregnancy is well tolerated with good control, precipitating factors should be avoided, and the need not to stop baseline medications for pregnancy. Spirometry is desirable to mark the baseline reference point and serial monitoring during pregnancy.[10]

Medication during Pregnancy

Asthma medication in pregnancy can be divided into:
- *Rescue medications:* Those required to provide symptomatic relief and treat bronchospasm like beta-2 agonist and ipratropium.
  - *Short-acting inhaled:* β2-adrenergic agonists—albuterol, isoproterenol,

pirbuterol metaproterenol, and terbutaline
- Inhaled anticholinergic agents ipratropium
- *Maintenance medication:* To control airway hyper-reactivity and treat underlying inflammation, like inhaled and systemic corticosteroids.

Apart from these leukotriene and cromolyn can be used.

Inhaled Corticosteroids

- *Low potency:* Beclomethasone dipropionate
- *Medium potency:* Triamcinolone acetonide
- *High potency:* Fluticasone propionate, budesonide, flunisolide, and mometasone furoate.

Inhaled corticosteroids are the most important pharmacologic agents in maintaining asthma control in and out of pregnancy.[11]

- *Mast cell stabilizers:* Disodium cromoglycate (cromolyn)
- *Leukotriene antagonists:* Zafirlukast, montelukast, and zileuton Theophylline, aminophylline.

Systemic Steroids

- *Oral:* Prednisone
- *Intravenous:* Methylprednisolone and hydrocortisone.

Nonfluorinated systemic steroids do not cross the placenta because of placental metabolism (the same is not true for betamethasone or dexamethasone).[12] Even in higher doses, the effect of hydrocortisone or prednisone on the fetus in terms of suppression of the hypothalamic pituitary-adrenal axis is minimal.

ASSESSING DRUG SAFETY IN PREGNANCY

A large population-based study done in 2013 had 15–20% increased risk of perinatal mortality, preeclampsia, and preterm delivery than those without asthma. This ratio changes with severity.

Current data of safety is based on the stepwise approach, addition of biologic in acute exacerbation needs evaluation.[13]

The Vaccines and Medications in Pregnancy Surveillance System (VAMPSS) was initiated in 2009, coordinated by the American Academy of Allergy, Asthma, and Immunology and includes three research arms and an independent advisory committee.[14] These arms being first mother to baby safety in antenatal period, second was to see congenital defects in baby, third for postpartum safety during lactation.

PRINCIPLES OF MANAGEMENT

- *Stepwise management:* Meant to assist, not replace individual patient needs.
- *Classify severity:* Peak expiratory flow (PEF) is percent of personal best; FEV1 is percent predicted.
- Control symptoms as quickly as possible then step down to the least medication necessary to maintain control.
- Provide education on self-management and controlling environmental factors that make asthma worse (e.g., allergens and irritants).

Acute Asthma Exacerbation[10]

- Place the patient on oxygen to keep oxygen saturation (SpO_2) >95%.
- Administer inhaled β2-adrenergic agonist until improvement is obtained or toxicity is noted, e.g., albuterol metered dose inhaler (MDI) with spacer three to four puffs or albuterol nebulizer every 10–20 minutes.
- If exacerbation is mild-to-moderate (i.e., FEV1 or PEF >50% predicted) initiate oral corticosteroids (i.e., prednisone 1 mg/kg)

TABLE 3: Classification and safety during pregnancy.[10]

Category	Criteria	Step therapy
Mild intermittent	• Symptoms up to twice a week and/or • Nighttime symptoms up to twice a month • PEFR >80% predicted and day-to-day variability <20%	• No daily treatment necessary • Inhaled β_2-adrenergic agonists as needed
Mild persistent	• Symptoms more than twice a week but not daily and/or • Nighttime symptoms more than twice a month • PEFR >80% predicted but day-to-day variability 20–30%	• Inhaled β_2-adrenergic agonists as needed and • Daily treatment with inhaled low-dose corticosteroid (preferably budesonide). • Alternatives include daily cromolyn, a leukotriene receptor antagonist, or a theophylline preparation
Moderate persistent	• Daily symptoms and/or • Nighttime symptoms more than once a week • PEFR 60–80% with day-to-day variability >30%	• Inhaled β_2-adrenergic agonists as needed and • Daily treatment with inhaled low-dose corticosteroid and daily treatment with salmeterol or • Daily treatment with inhaled medium-dose corticosteroid • If needed, combine treatment with daily medium-dose inhaled corticosteroid and daily salmeterol • Alternative: Daily low-medium dose inhaled corticosteroid and either theophylline or a leukotriene receptor antagonist
Severe persistent	• Continual symptoms that limit activity • Frequent nighttime symptoms and acute exacerbations • PEFR <60% predicted and day-to-day variability >30%	• Inhaled (β_2-adrenegic agonists as needed and • Daily treatment with inhaled high-dose corticosteroid and • Daily treatment with salmeterol and if needed • Daily treatment with systemic corticosteroids

Source: Adapted from Powrie RO. Drugs in pregnancy. Respiratory disease. Best Pract Res Clin Obstet Gynaecol. 2001;15:913-36.
(PEFR: peak expiratory flow rate)

- If exacerbation is severe (i.e., FEV1 or PEF <50% predicted) administer either oral or systemic steroids (e.g., methylprednisolone 125 mg IV acutely and then 40–60 mg IV 6 hourly or hydrocortisone 60–80 mg IV 6 hourly. When the patient improves, she can be switched to a tapering oral regimen of prednisone).
- Consider the use of ipratropium MDI (two puffs of 18 µg/spray q6h) or nebulizer (one 62.5 mL vial by nebulizer q6h) in the first 24 hours after the presentation.
- Initiate assessment of fetal well-being if pregnancy has reached fetal viability.
- Make an individualized assessment of the need for hospitalization.

Management in Intrapartum Period

Intrapartum period may be an associated factor for precipitating asthma, careful induction medications and continuation of inhalation bronchodilator are required. Oxytocin and prostaglandin E2 can be used to induce labor in asthmatics. Prostaglandin F2α (PGF2α) is contraindicated in pregnancy with asthma.[15]

General measures should include:
- Adequate analgesia will decrease the risk of bronchospasm.
- Women who are currently receiving or recently have taken systemic corticosteroids should receive intravenous administration of corticosteroids (e.g., hydrocortisone 100 mg every 8 hours) during labor and for 24 hours after delivery to prevent adrenal crisis.
- Acute exacerbation is not an indication for cesarean section.

Fetal Surveillance

The American College of Obstetricians and Gynecologists (ACOG) recommends that ultrasound examinations and antenatal fetal testing should be considered for women who have moderate or severe asthma during pregnancy.[15]
- First trimester ultrasound dating should be performed.
- Serial ultrasound examinations to monitor fetal activity and growth should be considered (starting at 32 weeks of gestation) for women who have poorly controlled asthma or moderate-to-severe asthma and for women recovering from a severe asthma exacerbation.

Management in Postnatal and Lactation

- Asthma medications continued postpartum
- PEFR to be monitored
- Breastfeeding is recommended in women regardless of their asthma treatment
- Chest physiotherapy

Barriers to asthma control: Women in pregnancy many a time avoid taking medication or stop taking if they were taking earlier due to many reasons. As per asthma knowledge, care, and outcome during pregnancy—the QAKCOP study analysis of 2019, fear of corticosteroids, side effects on the fetus, financial reasons, and inadequate follow-up in the prenatal period were identified as barrier to asthma control.[16]

Baseline improvement in patient education and adequate follow-up along with close association in management of physician and obstetrician are the keys to optimal management.

■ CONCLUSION

- The ultimate goal of asthma therapy in pregnancy is maintaining adequate oxygenation of the fetus by preventing hypoxic episodes in the mother.
- Step care approach—increase dose and medication according to severity.
- Inhaled corticosteroids are used for first-line control for persistent asthma during pregnancy.
- Identifying and controlling or avoiding factors such as allergens and irritants, particularly tobacco smoke, can lead to improved maternal well-being with less need for medication.[15]
- PFT assessment of patients during outpatient visits, spirometry is preferred, but PEF measurement with a peak flow meter is also sufficient.
- Even mild disease should be monitored with PEFR and FEV1 testing.
- Both maintenance and reduce medications should be used as a part of treatment.
- Use of prednisone, theophylline, antihistamines, inhaled corticosteroids, β_2-agonists, and cromolyn is not contraindicated for breastfeeding.

- Asthma self-management skills should include education and handling of worse signs and symptoms.

REFERENCES

1. World Health Organization. (2022). Asthma. [online] Available from https://www.who.int/news-room/fact-sheets/detail/asthma. [Last accessed April, 2023].
2. Aguilar R, Martinez J, Turcios E, Castro V. Asthma and pregnancy prevalence in a developing country and their mortality outcomes. J Pulmonol Respir Res. 2021; 5(1):88-93.
3. Shebl E, Chakraborty RK. Asthma in Pregnancy. Treasure Island (FL): StatPearls Publishing; 2023.
4. Chaouat G, Ledee-Bataille N, Dubanchet S, Zourbas S, Sandra O, Martal J. Reproductive immunology 2003: reassessing the Th1/Th2 paradigm? Immunol Lett. 2004;92(3):207-14.
5. Asthma.net. (2015). Classifying Asthma Severity. [online] Available from https://asthma.net/basics/classifications. [Last accessed April, 2023].
6. Arias F, Bhide A, Arulkumaran S, Damania K, Daftary S. Arias' Practical Guide to High-Risk Pregnancy and Delivery, 5th edition. Amsterdam, Netherlands: Elsevier; 2019.
7. Liccardi G, D'Amato M, D'Amato G. Asthma in pregnant patients: pathophysiology and management. Monaldi Arch Chest Dis. 1998;53(2):151 9.
8. Tamási L, Bohács A, Bikov A, Andorka C, Rigó J, Losonczy G, et al. Exhaled Nitric Oxide in Pregnant Healthy and Asthmatic Women. J Asthma. 2009;46(8):786-91.
9. Nathan RA, Sorkness CA, Kosinski M, Schatz M, Li JT, Marcus P, et al. Development of the asthma control test: a survey for assessing asthma control. J Allergy Clin Immunol. 2004;113(1):59-65.
10. James D, Steer P, Weiner C, Gonik B. (2005). High-Risk Pregnancy. [online] Available from https://openlibrary.org/books/OL34556337M/HighRisk_Pregnancy. [Last accessed April, 2023].
11. Martel MJ, Rey E, Beauchesne MF, Perreault S, Lefebvre G, Forget A, et al. Use of inhaled corticosteroids during pregnancy and risk of pregnancy induced hypertension: nested case–control study. BMJ. 2005;330(7485):230.
12. Schatz M, Zeiger RS, Harden K, Hoffman CC, Chilingar L, Petitti D. The safety of asthma and allergy medications during pregnancy. J Allergy Clin Immunol. 1997;100(3):301-6.
13. Chambers CD, Krishnan JA, Alba L, Albano JD, Bryant AS, Carver M, et al. The safety of asthma medications during pregnancy and lactation: Clinical management and research priorities. J Allergy Clin Immunol. 2021;147(6):2009-20.
14. Schatz M, Chambers CD, Jones KL, Louik C, Mitchell AA. Safety of influenza immunizations and treatment during pregnancy: the Vaccines and Medications in Pregnancy Surveillance System. Am J Obstet Gynecol. 2011;204(6 Suppl 1):S64-68.
15. Dombrowski MP, Schatz M; ACOG Committee on Practice Bulletins-Obstetrics. ACOG Practice Bulletin: clinical management guidelines for obstetrician-gynecologists number 90, February 2008: asthma in pregnancy. Obstet Gynecol. 2008;111(2 Pt 1): 457-64.
16. Ibrahim WH, Rasul F, Ahmad M, Bajwa AS, Alamlih LI, El Arabi AM, et al. Asthma knowledge, care, and outcome during pregnancy: The QAKCOP study. Chron Respir Dis. 2019;16:1479972318767719.

Heart Diseases in Pregnancy

Divya Agrawal

INTRODUCTION

Heart diseases (cardiac diseases) in the pregnant patient can present challenges in cardiovascular and maternal-fetal management.[1] Heart diseases of pregnancy encompasses a wide spectrum of pathologies. The complicated hormonal and physiological changes of pregnancy may lead of these disorders to manifest as new disease processes or they may exacerbate preexisting conditions that the pregnant women already have. Women who have preexisting illnesses such as hypertension, diabetes mellitus, and congenital heart disorders are more likely to develop cardiovascular disease.[2] Incidence of cardiac disease and pregnancies vary from 0.3 to 3.5%.[3]

Despite the high risk associated with these pregnancies, most of the cases can be effectively managed, if early diagnosis and thorough monitoring are part of standard medical care.

PATHOPHYSIOLOGY

Pregnancy is a natural stress and the significant morphological, physiological **(Table 1)**, and functional changes in cardiac physiology induced by pregnancy may have a significant impact on underlying heart disorders.

The women who have underlying cardiac disease might not always be able to adapt to these changes, and the ventricular dysfunction might result in cardiogenic heart failure. Due to the highest cardiac output, heart failure occurs frequently between 28 and 32 weeks. Cardiac failure in pregnant women with cardiac disease may precipitate during labor or the peripartum period and get worse with eclampsia, anemia, hemorrhage, and sepsis.

TABLE 1: Physiological changes in pregnancy.

Parameters in CVS	% changes during pregnancy
Cardiac output	Increase by 43%
Hart rate	Increase by 17%
Left ventricular work/index	Increase by 17%
Vascular resistance in systemic vessels	Decrease by 21%
Vascular resistance in pulmonary vessels	Decrease by 34%
MAP	Increase by 4%
Colloid osmotic pressure	Decrease by 14%

Source: Williams JW. Cardiovascular Disorders. In: Cunningham FG, Leveno KJ, Bloom SL, Dashe JS, Hoffman BL, Casey BM, Spong CY (Eds). Williams Obstetrics, 25th edition. New York, United States: McGraw Hill; 2018.
(CVS: cardiovascular system; MAP: mean arterial pressure)

RISK FACTORS FOR CARDIOVASCULAR DISEASE

- *Race/ethnicity:* Independent of other factors, non-Hispanic black women are

3.4 times more likely than non-Hispanic white women to die from cardiovascular disease-related pregnancy complications.
- *Age:* For women over 40 years, heart disease-related maternal mortality is 30 times more than for those under 20 years.
- *Hypertension:* Hypertensive diseases can cause maternal morbidity and mortality and impact up to 10% of pregnancies. Women are more at risk for cardiac impairment during or after delivery if they have early-onset and severe gestational hypertension.
- *Obesity:* Prepregnancy obesity raises the probability of maternal mortality due to heart diseases, especially if it is coupled with moderate-to-severe obstructive sleep apnea.
- Family history of heart disease.
- Addiction to alcohol, tobacco, and smoking.

The patient should be suspected of having maternal heart disease and pregnancy-related morbidity and mortality, if one or more of these risk factors are present **(Fig. 1)**.

DIAGNOSIS OF HEART DISEASES

Normal pregnancy's physiological changes can affect clinical findings and induce symptoms that could cloud the diagnosis of heart disease **(Table 2)**. As a crucial step toward enhancing maternal outcomes, healthcare professionals should know about the signs and symptoms **(Table 3)** of cardiovascular disease.[3]

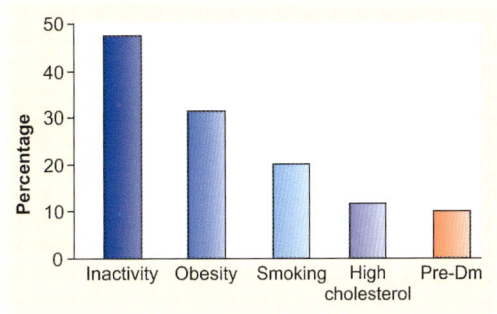

Fig. 1: Prevalence of cardiovascular disease risk factors in women of childbearing age. (DM: diabetes mellitus).
Source: Williams JW. Cardiovascular Disorders. In: Cunningham FG, Leveno KJ, Bloom SL, Dashe JS, Hoffman BL, Casey BM, Spong CY (Eds). Williams Obstetrics, 25th edition. New York, United States: McGraw Hill; 2018.

TABLE 2: Comparison of typical pregnancy symptoms and signs with abnormal pregnancy symptoms and signs indicative of cardiac disease.

	Routine care	*Caution*	*Stop*
	Reassurance	Nonemergent evaluation	Prompt evaluation pregnancy heart team
History of CVD	No	No	Yes
Self reported symptoms	None or mild	Yes	Yes
Shortness of breath		With new onset asthma, moderate exertion, persistent cough, or moderate or severe OSA	At rest; bilateral chest infiltrates on CXR or refectory pneumonia, paroxysmal nocturnal dyspnea or orthopnea
Chest pain	Reflux related which resolves with management	Atypical	At rest or with minimal exertion

Contd...

Contd...

	Routine care	Caution	Stop
Palpitation	Few second, self-limited	Brief, self-limited episodes; no syncope or light-headedness	Associated with near syncope
Syncope	Dizziness only with prolonged standing or dehydration	Vasovagal	Exertional or unprovoked
Fatigue vital signs	Mild normal	Mild or moderate	Extreme
HR (beats per minute)	<90	90–119	≥120
Systolic BP (mm Hg)	120–139	140–159	≥160 (or symptomatic low BP)
RR (per minute)	12–15	16–25	S2s
Oxygen saturation Physical examination	>97% Normal	95–97%	<95% (unless chronic)
JVP	Not visible	Not visible	Visible >2% cm above clavicle
Heart	S3, barely audible soft systolic murmur	S3, systolic murmur	Loud systolic murmur, diastolic murmur, S4
Lungs	Clear	Clear	Crackles, wheezing, effusion
Edema	Mild	Moderate	Marked

Source: American College of Obstetricians and Gynecologists' Presidential Task Force on Pregnancy and Heart Disease and Committee on Practice Bulletins—Obstetrics. ACOG Practice Bulletin No. 212: Pregnancy and Heart Disease. Obstet Gynecol. 2019;133(5):e320-56.
(BP: blood pressure; CVD: cardiovascular disease; CXR: chest X-ray; HR: heart rate; JVP: Jugular venous pressure; OSA: obstructive sleep apnea; RR: respiratory rate)

TABLE 3: Clinical indicators of cardiovascular disease in pregnancy.

Symptoms	Clinical findings

• Progressive dyspnea or orthopnea
• Nocturnal cough
• Hemoptysis
• syncope
	• Clubbing and cyanosis
	• Persistent neck vein enlargement
	• Grade 3/6 systolic murmur
	• Criteria for pulmonary hypertension:
	  – Diastolic murmur
	  – Persistent tachycardia
	  – Cardiomyopathy and arrhythmia
	  – Split-second heart sound

Source: Williams JW. Cardiovascular Disorders. In: Cunningham FG, Leveno KJ, Bloom SL, Dashe JS, Hoffman BL, Casey BM, Spong CY (Eds). Williams Obstetrics, 25th edition. New York, United States: McGraw Hill; 2018.

■ EVALUATION

It is frequently necessary to perform a thorough workup while evaluating the heart disease in pregnant women.

Diagnostic Investigation for Cardiac Disease in Pregnancy

- *Electrocardiogram (ECG):* It helps in diagnosis of almost all cardiac problems. However, following are the physiological changes during pregnancy:
  • Reduced mean PR interval
  • Increased heart rate
  • Left axis deviation
- *X-ray:*
  • It helps to diagnose cardiomegaly and pulmonary embolism

- Anteroposterior (AP) and lateral view
- Fetal exposure can be minimized when a lead apron shield is used
- Cardiomegaly can be excluded.
- *Echocardiography:*
  - Permits accurate diagnosis for cardiac problems
  - In few cases, transesophageal echo is useful.
- *Cardiac troponin I, troponin T, and "high-sensitivity" troponin:*
  - Sensitive and specific biomarkers of myocardial damage include cardiac troponin I, T, and "high-sensitivity" troponin.
  - The diagnosis of acute coronary syndrome during pregnancy includes symptoms which are similar to those in the general adult population, including abnormal ECGs, and increases in biomarkers such as troponin.
- *Natriuretic peptides:* N-terminal pro-brain natriuretic peptide (NT-proBNP) and brain natriuretic peptide (BNP) are natriuretic peptides. Natriuretic peptides should be measured in the presence of new clinical symptoms or signs suggestive of heart failure to prevent delayed diagnosis. Baseline BNP is advised in pregnant women who are at risk of or with known heart diseases, such as dilated cardiomyopathy and congenital heart diseases (CHDs).
- *Exercise stress test:* It is a crucial indicator of a woman's tolerance for pregnancy
- *D-dimer:* Not advised as a part of normal heart disease evaluation. It is primarily used for pulmonary embolism.
- *Angiography:* Coronary syndromes
- *CT/MRI:* For cardiomyopathies, aneurysms, etc.
- *Ultrasonography (USG):* Whenever indicated.

CLASSIFICATION OF FUNCTIONAL HEART DISEASE

For precisely assessing functional cardiac capacity, there is no therapeutically useful test. The clinical classification of the New York Heart Association (NYHA), initially published in 1928, is based on present and previous disability and is unaffected by physical signs:

- *Class I:*
  - *Uncompromised—no restrictions on physical activity:* These women do not exhibit any signs of heart insufficiency or feel angina pain.
- *Class II:*
  - *Slightly restricted physical activity:* At rest these women are comfortable, but when they engage in regular physical activity, they experience excessive fatigue, palpitations, dyspnea, or angina pain.
- *Class III:*
  - *Marked restriction of physical activity:* At rest these women are comfortable, but severe exhaustion, palpitations, dyspnea, or angina pain result from less than ordinary activity.
- *Class IV:*
  - *Significantly compromised—Unable to engage in any physical activity without experiencing discomfort*: Cardiac insufficiency or angina symptoms can appear even at rest. Discomfort increases with any physical exercise.

However, a revised classification of maternal cardiovascular risk has been established by the World Health Organization (WHO) **(Table 4)**. This is a tool used to assess the risk status of pregnant women with different types of preexisting cardiovascular diseases. The categories are listed in **Table 4**.

■ MANAGEMENT

Most of the times, management entails a collaborative effort by an obstetrician, cardiologist, anesthesiologist, and other experts as required. Early prenatal evaluation by a multidisciplinary team is advised for women with complex lesions or women who are particularly at risk.

Preconception Counseling

Women with severe heart diseases will benefit with counseling. Risk assessment,

TABLE 4: Modified World Health Organization (mWHO) pregnancy risk assessment classification for women with preexisting cardiovascular disease.

Modified WHO pregnancy risk classification (risk of pregnancy by medical conditions) Suggested follow-up	Specific cardiac lesions	Pregnancy care delivery location

mWHO risk class I:
No or only a slight increase in morbidity (2–5% risk of maternal cardiac event rate), and no discernible increase in the risk of maternal death
 	
Follow-up: Cardiology evaluation once or twice during pregnancy
	• Uncomplicated, small, or mild
	  – Patient ducts arteriosus
	  – Pulmonary stenosis
	  – Prolapse mitral valve
	• Successfully repaired simple lesions (ventricular or atrial septal defect, PDA, anomalous pulmonary venous drainage)
	• Atrial or ventricular ectopic beats, isolated
		• Prepregnancy/pregnancy counseling
		• Local hospital care
		• Delivery at local hospital

mWHO risk class II: Minimal increased risk of maternal mortality or moderate increase in morbidity (6–10% maternal cardiac event rate) Follow-up: Cardiology checkup every trimester	• Unoperated ventricular or • atrial septal defect • Repaired aortic coarctation or tetralogy of Fallot • Most arrhythmias (supraventricular arrhythmias) • Turner syndrome without congenital cardiac diseases	• Prepregnancy/pregnancy counseling • Consultation/counseling by pregnancy heart team • Local hospital care • Delivery at local hospital
mWHO risk classes II and III: Intermediate increased risk of maternal mortality or moderate-to-severe increase in morbidity (11–19% maternal cardiac event rate) Follow-up: Cardiology checks, every trimester	• Mild left ventricular impairment (EF >45%) • Hypertrophic cardiomyopathy • Native or bioprosthetic valve disease not considered mWHO risk class I or IV (mild mitral stenosis and moderate aortic stenosis) • Marfan or other HTAD syndrome without aortic dilation • Aorta <45 mm in bicuspid aortic valve pathology • Repaired coarctation without residua (non-Turner) • Atrioventricular septal defect	• Prepregnancy/pregnancy counseling • Pregnancy heart team consultation/counseling • Care at an appropriate level hospital (critical members of the pregnancy heart team available depending on cardiac disease) • Delivery at an appropriate level hospital

Contd...

Contd…

Modified WHO pregnancy risk classification (risk of pregnancy by medical conditions) Suggested follow-up	Specific cardiac lesions	Pregnancy care delivery location
Pre-mWHO risk class III: Significantly increased risk of maternal mortality or severe morbidity (20–27% maternal cardiac event rate) Follow-up: Cardiology, every 1–2 months	• Moderate left ventricular impairment (EF 30–45%) • Previous peripartum cardiomyopathy without any residual left ventricular impairment • Mechanical valve • Systemic right ventricle with good or mildly decreased ventricular function • Uncomplicated Fontan circulation • Unrepaired cyanotic heart disease • Severe asymptomatic aortic stenosis • Moderate mitral stenosis • Moderate aortic dilation (40–45 mm in Marfan syndrome or other HTAD; 45–50 mm in bicuspid aortic valve; Turner syndrome ASI 20–25 mm/m^2; tetralogy of Fallot < 50 mm) • Ventricular tachycardia • Other complex heart disease	• Prepregnancy/pregnancy counseling • Pregnancy heart team consultation/counseling • Care at an appropriate level hospital • Delivery at an appropriate level hospital
mWHO risk class IV: • Pregnancy contraindicated • Discuss-induced abortion • Extremely high risk of maternal mortality or severe morbidity (>27% maternal cardiac event rate) Follow-up: Cardiology follow-up every month (minimum)	• Pulmonary arterial hypertension • Severe systemic ventricular dysfunction (EF <30%, NYHA III-IV) • Previous peripartum cardiomyopathy with any residual left ventricular dysfunction • Severe mitral stenosis • Severe symptomatic aortic stenosis • Systemic right ventricle with moderate to severely decreased ventricular function • Severe aortic dilation (>45 mm in Marfan syndrome or other HTAD; >50 mm in bicuspid aortic valve; Turner syndrome ASI >25 mm/m^2; tetralogy of Fallot >50 mm) • Vascular Ehlers-Danlos • Severe (re)coarctation • Fontan circulation with any complication	• Pregnancy heart team consultation/counseling • Care at an appropriate level hospital (critical members of the pregnancy heart team available depending on cardiac disease) • Delivery at an appropriate level hospital

Source: American College of Obstetricians and Gynecologists' Presidential Task Force on Pregnancy and Heart Disease and Committee on Practice Bulletins—Obstetrics. ACOG Practice Bulletin No. 212: Pregnancy and Heart Disease. Obstet Gynecol. 2019;133(5):e320-56.
(EF: ejection fraction; HTAD: heritable thoracic aortic disease; NYHA: New York Heart Association; PDA: patent ductus arteriosus)

possible life-threating complications during pregnancy, and increased mortality have to be informed to the patient and relatives. All patients with cardiac disease to be properly assessed by cardiologist, physician, gynecologist, and risk assessed to be conveyed to the patient. Regular assessment of antenatal care (ANC) visit, hospitalization, complications, interventions, if required, depending on type of cardiac disease, their effect on pregnancy like prosthetic value replacement, and anticoagulant therapy should be explained. Contraceptive method to prevent unwanted pregnancy should also be discussed. Issues of CHD, i.e., increase risk or mortality and increase risk of CHD in offspring should be informed. Genetic Counseling of patient with Marfan syndrome and long QT syndrome have risk of inheritance of about 50%.

General Approaches to Pregnancy Management in Cardiac Patients

Antepartum Management Principles

- The resources required to reduce maternal and fetal difficulties should be anticipated, specified, and documented prior to delivery. Pregnant women with heart disease should give birth at a hospital with the appropriate maternal level of care.
- Smoking and alcohol should be prohibited.
- Frequent antenatal visits, i.e., every 2 weeks up to 28 weeks then every weekly up to delivery. NYHA class I and II patients are admitted 2 weeks before expected date of delivery (EDD) or if they develop any cardiac symptom during pregnancy. Class IV patients is continuously hospitalized while class III can take breaks from hospitalization if stable.
- Adequate rest is ensured. Excessive weight gain is avoided. Prevention; early detection; and treatment of anemia, infection, and hypertension should be done.
- Continue prophylaxis against recurrence of rheumatic fever, i.e., injection Penidure 2.4 mega units intramuscular (IM) every 3 weeks. Ensure endocarditis prophylaxis during any minor surgical procedure.
- Patients having high risk for mortality should be advised medical termination of pregnancy (MTP).

These include: (1) primary pulmonary hypertension (PHT), (2) Eisenmenger syndrome, (3) coarctation of aorta complicated, and (4) Marfan syndrome with aortic involvement. Relative indications include: (1) class III and IV diseases if family is completed, (2) severe aortic stenosis (AS), (3) cyanotic CHD, and (4) history of congestive cardiac failure (CCF) in previous pregnancy or in between pregnancy.

Intrapartum Management Principles

Vaginal delivery is preferred despite of the physical efforts required in labor as it has less morbidity and mortality. Induction of labor is avoided unless necessary. Cesarean section (CS) in reserved for obstetric indications or some other indications of CS includes dilated aortic root 4 cm or aortic aneurysm, acute severe CCF, recent myocardial infarction (MI), severe symptomatic AS, and need for emergency valve replacement surgery before delivery. However, in present times with better anesthetic facilities, newer cardiac drugs, and multipara monitors available CS is liberally done.

First stage:
- Supine position is avoided. Propped up semirecumbent position is the best.

- Oxygen therapy is given as required. Pulse oximetry should be done. Central venous pressure (CVP) monitoring is advisable.
- Nutrition is maintained by oral drinks. Intravenous (IV) fluid should be restricted to <60 mL/hour.
- Pulse, blood pressure (BP), respiration monitoring, and chest examination should be done every 30 minutes or more frequently if needed. Continuous ECG monitoring is advised and in case of PHT Swan-Ganz catheter to measure pulmonary capillary wedge pressure is advocated.
- Antibiotics prophylaxis against infective endocarditis is given by ampicillin or cephalosporin with gentamycin.
- For women receiving prophylactic heparin, cessation is advised at 12 hours prior to scheduled induction of labor or scheduled CS.[4]
- Pulmonary edema and arrhythmias are the most frequent intrapartum cardiac complications.[5] These patients need close monitoring and care.

Obstetric anesthesia principles: Patients with cardiac disease need a higher level of monitoring and anesthetic care during all obstetric procedures, including vaginal or cesarean deliveries. Antepartum consultation with an anesthesiologist is recommended for planning and assessing anesthetic, cardiac, and obstetric risks. Under the supervision of an anesthesiologist, patients with cardiac disease undergoing vaginal delivery should be advised epidural labor analgesia, and cardiac disease patients going for CS should be preferably offered neuraxial anesthesia. With the epidural use, cardiovascular events (often arrhythmia) are greatly reduced.[6] Contraindications for neuraxial anesthesia include the usual anesthetic contraindications and patients receiving anticoagulation.

Second stage: Lithotomy position should be avoided. Pulse and respiration are measured every 10 minutes. Outlet forceps (preferred) or vacuum should be used to shorten the second stage.

Third stage: Active management of third stage is not done. If there is atonic postpartum hemorrhage (PPH) concentrated oxytocin 20 units in IV drip or prostaglandin IM injection (carboprost) 250 µg is administered. Ergometrine is better avoided.

Postpartum Management Principles

Heart disease-related maternal morbidity and mortality are more likely to occur during the postpartum period than during any other time.[7]

The first 7 days after delivery and for up to 6 months following delivery are the most vulnerable times for immediate complications.[8]

This risk is increased by the co-occurrence of postpartum obstetric problems that arise immediately after delivery, such as hypertensive disorders, hemorrhage, and infection.

Careful observation is must as heart failure can occur immediate postpartum (sudden additional bloodload from the uterus) or later (mobilization of extravascular fluid in the vascular system).

Adequate bed rest with gentle leg exercises and breathing exercise is advocated to prevent thromboembolic and chest complications. Breastfeeding is allowed except in patient with heart failure. Breastfeeding has favorable effect on maternal hypertension and maternal vasculature.

Contraception:
Permanent: Vasectomy is preferred to female sterilization. In female, minilaparotomy tubal ligation (TL) under local anesthesia after at least 1 week of delivery or interval laparoscopic TL using less gas and less head low position can be the option.

Temporary: Oral pills are avoided due to risk of thromboembolism; progestogen-only contraceptives can be used. Intrauterine contraceptive device (IUCD) is avoided due to risk of infection. Barrier method is the method of choice but high failure rate is a problem.

Special Cardiac Conditions

Valvular Heart diseases

Mitral stenosis: Most of mitral stenosis cases are due to rheumatic endocarditis, and pregnant women are at a significant risk of morbidity and mortality due to the obstructive nature of mitral stenosis.[9] Beta-blockers continue to be the drug of choice even though; no drugs have been demonstrated to reverse this condition in these patients. It is believed that beta-blockers reduce the transmitral gradient. For the treatment of heart failure, diuretics are helpful.

Women having severe mitral stenosis may need surgical intervention.

Aortic stenosis: Despite being less frequent, AS in pregnancy is often more challenging to treat. It is necessary to strictly restrict the activity. When it comes to lowering the transvalvular gradient, beta-blockers are not as useful as in mitral stenosis. Ace inhibitors should not be used on pregnant patients. Due to the possibility of decreased diastolic filling and further decreased cardiac output, diuretic medication should be used with caution.

Mitral Regurgitation and Aortic Regurgitation

As the systemic vascular resistance decrease and the forward flow increase in pregnancy, these are tolerated during pregnancy.

Pulmonary and Tricuspid Valve Diseases

These are rare and usually well tolerated.

Peripartum Cardiomyopathy

Diagnostic criteria suggested by Demakis and Rahimmtoola[10] include:
- Heart failure in the last month of pregnancy or 5 months after delivery
- No history of previous heart illness
- No known etiology of heart failure
- Echocardiography shows left ventricular dysfunction echo changes suggested by Hibbard et al.[11] It include:
  - Ejection fraction <45%
  - Fractional shortening <30%
  - Left ventricle end-diastolic dimension >2.7cm/m^2.

Fatigue, dyspnea with exertion, orthopnea, generalized chest pain, peripheral edema, and discomfort in the abdomen are common clinical symptoms. Although rare, it carries high risk of mortality, i.e., 25–50%. It is found more in patients with hypertension, multiple pregnancy, and increased maternal age and parity. There is no recognized cause for peripartum cardiomyopathy (PPCM). Heart failure is managed in the usual manner. Medical treatment for PPCM may be stared during pregnancy and continued after delivery. Hydralazine, digoxin, and diuretics can all be administered without risk throughout pregnancy and while nursing. Beta-blockers may enhance left ventricular function in these patients. Women with PPCM may need intense IV therapy, mechanical assist devices, or possibly heart transplantation when standard medical treatment is ineffective. Future pregnancy is not recommended due to the significant probability of recurrence.

Congenital Heart Diseases

- *Left-to-right shunts:* Pregnancy is often well tolerated by atrial septal defect (ASD), ventricular septal defect (VSD), and patent ductus arteriosus (PDA) patients. The primary factor that determines the degree of disability is the size of the defect.

- *Coarctation of aorta:* It is uncommon in women and it is frequently related with bicuspid aortic valve and cerebral artery aneurysms. Risks of cerebral hemorrhage, infectious endocarditis, and aortic dissection are increased during pregnancy. CS is indicated only for obstetric reasons.
- *Tetralogy of Fallot:* It includes pulmonary stenosis, right ventricular hypertrophy, a large VSD, and an overriding of the aorta. Pregnancy is poorly tolerated in those who have not undergone surgical repair, so MTP is recommended.
- *Marfan syndrome:* It has an autosomal dominant inheritance. Due to myxomatous degeneration of heart valves and cystic medical necrosis of the aorta there is increased chances of aneurysms. Pregnancy is highly risky in such cases because of aortic dissection and rupture.
- *Pulmonary stenosis:* Usually well tolerated during pregnancy. In severe stenosis congestive heart failure can occur.
- *Eisenmenger syndrome:* It is characterized by PHT secondary to right-to-left or bidirectional stunt because of high maternal and perinatal mortality (severe maternal hypoxemia and polycythemia). MTP is advised.
- *Idiopathic hypertrophic subaortic stenosis (IHSS):* There is marked hypertrophy of ventricular septum leading to outflow obstruction. Hypervolemia should be avoided.

Pulmonary Hypertension

There is high maternal mortality rate, 30–50% in pulmonary arterial hypertension and Eisenmenger syndrome. Maternal deaths occur in last trimester of pregnancy and first month after delivery because of PHT crisis or pulmonary embolism. Management of PHT includes counseling for avoiding pregnancy and MTP if pregnancy occurs. If she wants to continue pregnancy, delivery under cardiac consultation should be done either lower segment cesarean section (LSCS) or normal vaginal delivery at higher center associated with cardiac facility.

Pregnant Woman with Prosthetic Valves

Bioprosthetic valve do not require anticoagulation during pregnancy. But due to short life of such valves mechanical prostatic valves are now used, which require lifelong anticoagulation.

Anticoagulants:

Warfarin: Although warfarin freely crosses the placental barrier and may be harmful to the fetus, it is safe to use during breastfeeding. Warfarin embryopathy (defects in the development of fetal bone and cartilage), incidence is only 4–10%, with the risk being highest when it is given between 6 and 12 weeks of gestation.

Unfractionated heparin: Unfractionated heparin (UFH) is safe for the fetus as it does not cross the placenta. However, its use has been linked to a significant incidence of hemorrhage, maternal osteoporosis, thrombocytopenia, or thrombosis (heparin-induced thrombocytopenia and thrombosis, or HITT syndrome). The starting dose adjustment for UFH is based on an activated partial thromboplastin time (aPTT) of two to three times the control level. It is used subcutaneously. Heparin is stopped as soon as labor pains begin or 6 hours before elective CS, and it is restarted 6–12 hours after delivery.

Low-molecular-weight heparin: Compared to UFH, low-molecular-weight heparin (LMWH) exhibits a more consistent anticoagulant response and is less likely to result in HITT.

Warfarin should be stopped once the pregnancy is diagnosed, and UFH or LMWH should be used instead, at least after the 12th week.

Cardiac Arrhythmias

Significant cardiac arrhythmias are rare during pregnancy. Management of arrhythmias is similar to that in the nonpregnant stage. However, drugs that appear to be safe to use in pregnant women with tachyarrhythmias include adenosine, verapamil, digoxin, flecainide, and beta-blockers.[12] Exceptions are amiodarone which can cause neonatal hypothyroidism and sotalol which can cause fetal intrauterine growth restriction (IUGR).

Spontaneous Coronary Artery Dissection (SCAD)

This is an atypical cause of acute MI. Its incidence, however, increases in pregnant women. Spontaneous coronary artery dissection (SCAD) should be considered in any pregnant female presenting with symptoms consistent with acute coronary syndrome.[13] This dissection usually affects the left main or the left anterior descending artery. Diagnosis may be made using coronary angiography. Management, however, has not been standardized due to its rarity. Many different management strategies have been utilized. These include heart transplantation, coronary artery bypass grafting (CABG), or medical management.[14]

Coronary Artery Diseases

Acute myocardial infarction (AMI) during pregnancy is rare, occurring in 1 in 35,000 pregnancies. Angiotensin-converting enzyme (ACE) inhibitors and statins are contraindicated during pregnancy. Clopidogrel and glycoprotein IIb/IIIa receptor inhibitors have been used safely in individual pregnant patients. Percutaneous coronary interventions using both balloon angioplasty and stenting has been successfully performed in pregnant patients with AMI, with the use of lead shielding to protect the fetus.

Different scoring systems for predicting adverse outcome during pregnancy or are CARPREG I and II scoring and ZAHARA prediction score.

According to CARPREG I score[5] **(Table 5)**, risk estimation of cardiovascular complications is 5% if there is 0 point. It is 27% if there is one risk factor and it increase to 75% if there is more than one risk factor.

CARPREG II score[15] **(Table 6)** include 10 risk factors. Risk of cardiac event is 5% if score is 1, 10% if score is 2, 15% if score is 3, 22% if score is 4, and 41% if score is >4.

ZAHARA Prediction score[7] has been described in **Table 7**.

TABLE 5: Risk factors to estimate the risk of cardiac complications during pregnancy (CARPREG score)

Cardiac risk factor	Points
1. Prior heart failure, TI attacks, arrhythmia, and stroke	1
2. NYHA >II and cyanosis	1
3. Ejection fraction <40%	1
4. Left-sided heart obstruction, i.e., mitral <2 cm² Aortic valve <1.5 cm² or peak left ventricular outflow tract gradient >30 mm on echo	1

(NYHA: New York Heart Association; TI: transient ischemic)

TABLE 6: CARPREG II score.

Predictor	Point
1. Prior cardiac event or arrhythmias	3
2. Baseline NYHA >2 or cyanosis	3
3. Mechanical valve	3
4. Systemic ventricular dysfunction LVEF <55%	2
5. High-risk value disease or left ventricular outflow tract obstruction (aortic valve area <1.5 cm^2, subaortic gradient >30, or moderate-to-severe aortic regurgitation mitral stenosis <2.0 cm^2)	2
6. Pulmonary hypertension RVSP >49 mm Hg	2
7. High-risk aortopathy	2
8. Coronary artery disease	2
9. No prior cardiac intervention	1
10. Late pregnancy assessment	1

(LVEF: left ventricular ejection fraction; NNHYA: New York Heart Association; RSVP: right ventricular systolic pressure)

TABLE 7: ZAHARA prediction score.

Predictor	Point	Total points	Risk
Prior arrhythmias	1.5	0	2.9%
NYHA Class ≥2	0.75	0.5–1.5	17.5%
Left heart obstruction (PG >50 mm Hg or AVA <1 cm^2)	2.5	1.51–2.50	43%
Cardiac medication before pregnancy	1.5	2.51–3.50	43.1
Systemic AV value regurgitation	0.75	>3.51	70%
Pulmonary AV valve regurgitation	0.75		

(AV: atrioventricular; AVA: aortic valve area; NYHA: New York Heart Association)

■ COMPLICATIONS

Complications associated to heart disease in pregnancy include:
- Excessive weight gain during pregnancy
- Gestational hypertension
- Restricted intrauterine growth
- Preterm birth
- Abruptio placentae
- Hemorrhage
- Gestational diabetes
- Progressive heart failure
- Maternal or fetal demise.

Even though heart disease during pregnancy is a high-risk condition, patients who receive regular follow-up can experience excellent outcome. However, some pregnancy-related disorders are more likely to cause morbidity and mortality than others.

■ CONCLUSION

- Women with inherited or acquired heart conditions and aortic disorders should be evaluated for pregnancy risk and given counseling.

- All women with heart disease who are of reproductive age and after pregnancy should undergo risk assessment, according to the WHO.
- High-risk patients should be treated by a multidisciplinary team in a specialized facility.
- CHD patients should be advised genetic counseling.
- Etiology for congenital heart lesion is multifactorial and include genetic, diabetes, systemic lupus erythematosus (SLE), infections, e.g., rubella and alcohol ingestion.
- Risk of transmission to fetus in case of CHDs varies from 2 to 20%. In fetuses with increased nuchal translucency of >95th centile, 2% will have major cardiac defect.
- ECG, echo, and MRI must be performed in case of appearance of new symptomatic patient.
- Prevention of bacterial endocarditis must be followed.
- If the medical treatment is ineffective, cardiac bypass and valvular surgery may be explored.
- In most patients with heart diseases, vaginal delivery is the first choice.
- Breastfeeding is generally not contraindicated.
- Postpartum period must be followed up meticulously, especially high-risk heart disease cases.
- Decision regarding appropriate contraception method must be offered to the patient, vasectomy is the best option.
- In women on beta-blockers, there is increase change of IUGR.

REFERENCES

1. Warnes CA, Williams RG, Bashore TM, Child JS, Connolly HM, Dearani JA, et al. ACC/AHA 2008 Guidelines for the Management of Adults with Congenital Heart Disease: Executive Summary: a report of the American College of Cardiology/American Heart Association Task Force on Practice Guidelines (writing committee to develop guidelines for the management of adults with congenital heart disease). Circulation. 2008;118(23):2395-451.
2. Goldstein SA, Ward CC. Congenital and Acquired Valvular Heart Disease in Pregnancy. Curr CardiolRep. 2017;19(10):96.
3. Mosca L, Benjamin EJ, Berra K, Bezanson JL, Dolor RJ, Lloyd-Jones DM, et al. Effectiveness-based guidelines for the prevention of cardiovascular disease in women—2011 update: a guideline from the American Heart Association. Circulation. 2011;123(11):1243-62.
4. American College of Obstetricians and Gynecologists' Committee on Practice Bulletins—Obstetrics. ACOG Practice Bulletin No. 196: Thromboembolism in pregnancy. Obstet Gynecol. 2018;132:e1-17.
5. Siu SC, Sermer M, Colman JM, Alvarez AN, Mercier LA, Morton BC, et al. Prospective multicentre study of pregnancy outcomes in women with heart disease. Cardiac Disease in Pregnancy (CARPREG) Investigators. Circulation. 2001;104:515-21.
6. Tanaka H, Kamiya C, Katsuragi S, Tanaka K, Yoshimatsu J, Ikeda T. Effect of epidural anaesthesia in labor; pregnancy with cardiovascular disease. Taiwan J Obstet Gynecol. 2018;57:190-3.
7. Regitz-Zagrosek V, Roos-Hesselink JW, Bauersachs J, Blomstrom-Lundqvist C, Cifkova R, De Bonis M, et al. 2018 ESC guidelines for the management of cardiovascular diseases during pregnancy. ESC Scientific Document Group. Eur Heart J. 2018;39:3165-241.
8. ACOG Committee Opinion No. 736: Optimizing postpartum care. Obstet Gynecol. 2018;131:e140-50.
9. Silversides CK, Colman JM, Sermer M, Siu SC. Cardiac risk in pregnant women with rheumatic mitralstenosis. Am J Cardiol. 2003;91(11):1382-5.

10. Adamson DL, Nelson-Piercy C. Managing palpitations and arrhythmias during pregnancy. Heart. 2007;93(12):1630-6.
11. Bac DJ, Lotgering FK, Verkaaik AP, Deckers JW. Spontaneous coronary artery dissection during pregnancy and post partum. Eur Heart J. 1995;16(1):136-8.
12. Lane JE, Cartledge RG, Johnson JH. Successful surgical treatment of spontaneous coronary artery dissection. Curr Surg. 2001;58(3):316-8.
13. Demakis JG, Rahimtoola SH, Peripartum cardiomyopathy. Circulation. 1971;4:964-8.
14. Hibbard JU, Lindheimer M, Lang RM. A modified definition for peripartum cardiomyopathy and prognosis based on echocardiography. Obstet Gynecol. 1999;94(2):311-6.
15. Silversides CK, Grewal J, Mason J, Sermer M, Kiess M, Rychel V, et al. Pregnancy outcomes in women with heart diseases. The CARPREG II study. J Am Call Cardiol. 2018;71(21):2419-30.

Chapter 8

Liver Diseases in Pregnancy

Shweta Kumari

■ INTRODUCTION

There is progressive, anatomical, physiological, and biochemical change during pregnancy which is not only confined to genital organ but also to other organs of the body. Approximately 3% of pregnant women are affected by some form of liver diseases during pregnancy. Some of these can be fatal for both mother and child.[1]

The causes of liver diseases during pregnancy can be grouped as shown in **Table 1**.[1]

■ VIRAL HEPATITIS

Viral hepatitis is the most common cause of jaundice in pregnancy the pathogens responsible for viral hepatitis are hepatitis A, B, C, and E viruses, Epstein–Barr virus, herpes simplex virus, and human immunodeficiency virus. The highest maternal mortality is associated with hepatitis E virus while hepatitis B virus is associated with the maximum risk of vertical transmission and subsequently persistent chronic infection.

Hepatitis A Virus (Ribonucleic Acid Virus)

Transmission—feco-oral route.

T cell-mediated immune response is responsible for underlying pathogenesis thus this infection provides lifelong immunity.[2] Analysis is made by detecting serum anti-hepatitis A virus (HAV) immunoglobulin M (IgM) antibodies. Prevention is by improving the sanitary conditions and vaccinating the high-risk pregnant woman.[3-5] Treatment is symptomatic, improvement in sanitation and adequate nutrition.

TABLE 1: Classification of liver diseases in pregnancy.[1]

Liver diseases specific to pregnancy	Liver diseases concurrent to pregnancy
Intrahepatic cholestasis of pregnancy	Viral hepatitis
Severe preeclampsia, eclampsia, and HELLP syndrome	Gall stones (cholelithiasis)
Acute fatty liver of pregnancy	Drug-induced (anti-TB drug, antiepileptic drug, antiretroviral drug, and NSAIDs)
Severe hyperemesis gravidarum	Hemolytic jaundice
	Primary biliary cirrhosis and primary sclerosing cholangitis

(HELLP: hemolysis, elevated liver enzymes, and low platelets; NSAIDs: nonsteroidal anti-inflammatory drugs; TB: tuberculosis)

Hepatitis B Virus (Deoxyribonucleic Acid Virus)

Transmission—vertical transmission as well as horizontal transmission through sexual contact, transfusion through blood products, and parenteral route.

Acute infection is manifested by flu-like illness as malaise, abdominal pain, nausea, vomiting, tiredness, muscle and joint pain, jaundice, and sometimes fever. Neonatal transmission occurs mostly around time of birth. Approximately 25% of the carrier neonate die from liver cirrhosis or hepatic carcinoma between late childhood to early adulthood. Nearly 90% of patients clear the infection and have full recovery. 1% develop fulminant hepatitis. 10% become chronic cases. Analysis is made by liver function tests (LFTs) and serological detection of hepatitis B surface antigen (HBsAg), hepatitis B e antigen (HBeAg), antibody to hepatitis B core antigen (HBcAg), and hepatitis B virus (HBV) deoxyribonucleic acid (DNA) titer. Liver enzymes are elevated during initial phase. Universal screening with HBsAg is recommended at the first antenatal visit regardless of previous vaccination.[3,6] Once a pregnant women is tested HBV positive, the World Health Organization recommends testing for hepatitis D virus as coinfection can result in increased mortality. Counseling and screening of close contacts are also recommended.[4] Universal vaccination of all infants has played an important role in decreasing global burden.[3] High viral load (HBV DNA >10^6 copies/mL or >200,000 IU/mL) and high infectivity proven by envelope antigen (HBeAg) are responsible for this ineffective immunoprophylaxis,[5] and therefore these two tests should be done in the third trimester of all HBsAg positive cases.

Tenofovir (300 mg/dL) is the first-line drug, while telbivudine (600 mg/d, moderate resistance) and lamivudine (100 mg/d high resistance) can be used by starting at 28–30 weeks till 3 months postpartum (grade 2 B).[6] To reduce mother-to-child transmission (MTCT), one should avoid invasive procedures such as amniocentesis and internal electronic fetal monitoring during labour.[2] Pregnant woman who is seronegative should have hepatitis B immunoglobulin (HBIG) 0.06 mL/kg intramuscular (IM) soon following exposure and a second dose after 1 month. Then she should also be given recombinant DNA vaccine intramuscularly 1 mL, three doses at 0, 1, and 6 months interval. All infants born to HBsAg positive mother should get HBIG 0.5 mL IM within 12 hours of birth. Active immunization with hepatitis B vaccine (0.5 mL) is also given IM at separate sites. This is very effective to prevent neonatal infection.

Hepatitis C Virus (Ribonucleic Acid Virus)

The route of infection is the same as that of HBV with 60% chance of persisting to chronic hepatitis, out of them 20% have chance of developing cirrhosis and hepatocellular carcinoma. The risk of vertical transmission is 3–5%.[3] The Centers for Disease Control and Prevention (CDC) endorses anti-HCV testing for pregnant females with a high risk for infection.[6-9] Similar to HBV invasive techniques such as amniocentesis and internal electronic fetal monitoring should be avoided to reduce MTCT.[2]

Hepatitis E Virus (Ribonucleic Acid Virus)

Transmission—feco-oral route.

It may lead to fulminant hepatitis. Maternal mortality is high up to 20%. Infection is diagnosed by detecting IgM antibodies. Improving sanitation and avoiding travel to endemic areas prevent this infection.

■ AUTOIMMUNE HEPATITIS

This is an infective and progressive liver disease that can manifest anytime during pregnancy and postpartum. This is concomitant with prematurity, low-birth-weight baby, and fetal loss.

INTRAHEPATIC CHOLESTASIS OF PREGNANCY

The incidence of intrahepatic cholestasis of pregnancy (ICP) is between 0.2 and 2%. Risk factors for ICP include multiple gestation, in vitro fertilization, advanced maternal age, history of prior affected pregnancy, family history, and hepatitis C infection.[8,10,11] Women with ICP are more likely to develop hepatobiliary diseases, including fibrosis, gallstone diseases, and hepatitis.[10,11] Bile stasis occurs due to excess circulating estrogen. There is rise in conjugated bilirubin, alanine transaminase (ALT), aspartate transaminase (AST), and serum alkaline phosphatase. Bilirubin rarely exceeds 5 mg%. Onset is insidious. Symptoms are jaundice, pruritus, weakness, nausea, and vomiting. Obstetric cholestasis typically affects palms and soles, worsens at night.[12] Once diagnosed, the LFT should be measured weekly until delivery. Symptoms and biochemical parameters resolute after delivery, which secures diagnosis of obstetric cholestasis. Ursodeoxycholic acid (UDCA) is the drug of choice, can be given at dose of 300–600 mg daily orally. Literature suggests that 73–90% of acute cholecystitis responds to medical management in pregnancy.[13,14]

Topical emollients, calamine lotion, provides relief from pruritus and can be used safely in pregnancy. Stillbirth/fetal death are major concern involved with cholestasis. It is frequently sudden without any evidence of placental vascular insufficiency, intrauterine growth restriction, and oligohydramnios; therefore, Doppler, cardiotocography, biophysical profile, fetal movement count, etc., measures are not helpful in predicting fetal death. There is increased likelihood of meconium passage, preterm delivery, fetal distress, more cesarean incidences, and postpartum hemorrhage (PPH).[15-18] Injection vitamin K given prophylactically to reduce the chances of PPH. Postnatal vitamin K is given to neonate to prevent bleeding. It has high recurrence rate (45–90%) with family preponderance.

CIRRHOSIS AND PORTAL HYPERTENSION

Portal hypertension usually worsens in pregnancy. All cirrhotic patients should undertake variceal screening in the second trimester.[8]

Banding before pregnancy may be suitable for high risk varices. The greatest risk is seen in the second trimester and during delivery because of Valsalva maneuver.[19,20] Each episode of variceal bleeding carries maternal mortality rates as high as 20–50%.[8] LFT will be deranged along with hypoalbuminemia, raised prothrombin time (PT), and thrombocytopenia. Sonography with Doppler study may be helpful in advanced stage of disease. Management of variceal bleeding focuses on endoscopic variceal ligation and supportive care for mother and fetus.[21,22] Octreotide along with antibiotics appears to be a safe option as an adjunct treatment in acute bleeding.[8] Patients with cirrhosis have 10% risk of postpartum hemorrhage that may be associated with coagulopathy and thrombocytopenia due to hyperspleenism.[21] Cesarean delivery carries increased risk of bleeding complications in women with Pulmonary hypertension.[8] Therefore, vaginal delivery with shortened second stage has been advocated.[8,23] Elective termination of pregnancy can be considered in women with severe hepatic decompensation and liver failure.[21]

GALLSTONES/CHOLELITHIASIS IN PREGNANCY

The most common surgical problem associated with pregnancy is gallstone. Mostly they are asymptomatic. Even though some pregnant patients experience uncomplicated cholelithiasis, some develops complications such as acute cholecystitis, choledocholithiasis, cholangitis, and gallstone pancreatitis.[24] Both medical and surgical options for management are there. Asymptomatic cases are advised lifestyle changes and dietary modifications. Acute cholecystitis treated conservatively with intravenous (IV) fluids, antibiotics, antispasmodics, and bowel rest, but recurrence rate is high. For such cases second trimester is time to undergo surgery (cholecystectomy).

ACUTE FATTY LIVER OF PREGNANCY

It is the condition where fatty infiltration of liver occurs which can even lead to liver failure.[6] Prevalence of acute fatty liver of pregnancy (AFLP) is 1 in 15,000 pregnancies. This is an uncommon but potentially fatal disease unique to pregnancy that typically occurs after 30 weeks of gestation.[8,25,26] High risk groups are old primigravidas, multiple gestation, preeclamptic, and history of AFLP. Symptoms are anorexia, malaise nausea, vomiting, headache, pain in abdomen, ascites, and jaundice. Sometimes hypertension and disseminated intravascular coagulation (DIC) may be associated. Undiagnosed cases develop acute renal failure, hepatic encephalopathy, and mortality. AFLP and HELLP syndrome are coexistent in approximately 50% of patients.[8,25,27] Diagnosis made by elevations in liver enzymes, ALT, AST, bilirubin, blood urea nitrogen, uric acid, creatinine, leukocytosis, thrombocytopenia, hypoglycemia, and coagulopathy. Such cases need hospitalization and immediate delivery. Supportive measures as glucose infusion and others based on investigation report are given. Vaginal delivery is preferred as cesarean section increases morbidity. The condition improves after delivery with normal liver function within a week or two. Major causes of mortality are PPH, renal failure, hypoglycemia, DIC, pulmonary edema, and hepatic encephalopathy.[28,29]

LIVER TRANSPLANT

Pregnancy should be delayed for at least 1 year after liver transplantation. Although 70% of grafted women will deliver healthy baby.[1] Apart from the risk of infection following immune suppression, pregnancy after a transplant has a higher risk of chronic hypertension, preeclampsia, preterm delivery, premature rupture of membrane (PROM), and anemia.[30]

The fetal risks of exposure to cyclosporine, tacrolimus, azathioprine, sirolimus, everolimus, and corticosteroids appear to be low and the consequences of acute cellular rejection or graft loss with their discontinuation pose a much grave prognosis.[8] Corticosteroids are safe in pregnancy but can lead to fetal adrenal axis suppression, fetal growth restriction, and PROM.[31] Consultation with a maternal-fetal medicine specialist must be taken.

Mode of delivery planned based on obstetric condition. Congenital cytomegalovirus (CMV) infection can lead to neonatal death.

■ HYPEREMESIS GRAVIDARUM

Hyperemesis is severe type of vomiting of pregnancy which has got harmful effect on the health of the mother and disables her in day-to-day activities. Adverse effects which can be seen are dehydration, metabolic acidosis, metabolic alkalosis, electrolyte imbalance, and weight loss. The incidence is 0.3–2%.[32] Vomiting corresponds with the human chorionic gonadotropin (hCG) levels and commonly starts at fifth week, peaks at tenth week (when hCG levels are maximum), and usually disappears at around 16–18 weeks.[33] If not treated in time, it can cause fatty degeneration and necrosis of liver, esophageal perforation, Wernicke's encephalopathy, coma, seizures, and acute kidney injury. The high risk groups are obese, twin pregnancy, trophoblastic disease nulliparity, and history of hyperemesis in previous pregnancy.

Diagnosis is clinical and includes symptoms as nausea, vomiting, anxiety, sleep disturbances, and depression. Investigations done to assess the need for hospitalization are check vitals, LFT, kidney function test, and serum electrolytes. Ultrasound is done to rule out hydatidiform mole and multiple gestation. Management is to keep patient nil per orally with some fluids, multivitamin injections, and injectable antiemetics (ondansetron and metoclopramide). Once acute vomiting stops diet is gradually increased. The Food and Drug Administration (FDA) approved drug for pregnancy is a combination of pyridoxine and doxylamine. Hydrocortisone 100 mg IV in drip is given in case of hypotension or in intractable vomiting.

■ HELLP SYNDROME

This is the complicated form of liver abnormality seen in approximately 20% cases of severe preeclampsia or eclampsia.[34] It must be differentiated from hemolytic uremic syndrome (HUS), thrombotic thrombocytopenic purpura, and AFLP. It is associated with raised blood pressure, nausea, headache, epigastric pain, vomiting, jaundice, and elevated liver enzymes. Careful assessment of maternal and fetal status followed by delivery is the management protocol. Cesarean section is most common mode of delivery. Platelet transfusion given if required. Patient should be managed in intensive care unit (ICU) until there is improvement in platelet count, urine output, controlled blood pressure, and liver enzymes. Perinatal mortality ranges between 5 and 60% and maternal mortality may be up to 25%.

Maternal complications include abruptio placenta, DIC, acute renal failure, severe ascites, pulmonary edema, pleural effusion, cerebral edema retinal detachment, subcapsular liver hematoma, acute respiratory distress syndrome (ARDS), sepsis, and death. Perinatal morbidity and mortality is increased due to preterm delivery, ARDS, and sepsis. Differential diagnosis of jaundice during pregnancy has been provided in **Table 2**.[8]

TABLE 2: Differential diagnosis of jaundice during pregnancy.[8]

Reports	HELLP	AFLP	TTP	HUS
Jaundice (%)	5–10%	40–90%	Rare	Rare
Urine	Proteinuria	Proteinuria	Proteinuria	Proteinuria
Decrease thrombocyte	+	+	+	+
Hemolysis (%)	50–100%	15–20%	100%	100%
Anemia	Mild	No	Yes	Yes
DIC (%)	<20%	50–100%	Uncommon	Uncommon
Hypoglycemia	No	Common	No	No
Transaminase	High	High	Mild	Mild
Elevated bilirubin	Sometimes	Always	Always	Always
Reduced renal function (%)	50%	90–100%	30%	100% raised
Management	Delivery and recovery	Delivery and recovery	Plasma infusion or exchange	Plasma infusion or exchange

(AFLP: acute fatty liver of pregnancy; DIC: disseminated intravascular coagulation; HELLP: hemolysis, elevated liver enzyme, and low platelet count; HUS: hemolytic uremic syndrome; TTP: thrombotic thrombocytopenic purpura)

CONCLUSION

- Overall approximately 3% of total pregnancies are complicated by liver disorders.
- There is no histological change in liver cells but the functions are decreased due to mild cholestasis.
- Universal vaccination of all infants has contributed in lessening global burden of hepatitis B infection.
- All infants born to HBsAg positive mother should get HBV vaccine and HBIG within 12 hours of delivery.
- Breastfeeding is not contraindicated in mother having hepatitis.
- Maternal mortality is high in hepatitis E virus infection approximately up to 20%.
- Universal screening of hepatitis B and hepatitis C virus infection in pregnancy is suggested.
- Women having ICP are more likely to develop hepatobiliary diseases including fibrosis, gallstone diseases, and hepatitis.
- 73–90% cases of acute cholecystitis responds to medical management in pregnancy.
- Injection vitamin K given prophylactically to reduce PPH in liver diseases in pregnancy.
- Autoimmune hepatitis cases should continue steroid treatment with immunosuppressive drug in pregnancy.
- AFLP is uncommon but potentially fatal disease exclusive to pregnancy that typically occurs after 30 weeks of gestation.
- The clinical sign of hyperemesis gravidarum are due to starvation, dehydration, and ketoacidosis.
- Subcapsular liver hematoma is a life-threatening condition and occurs in 0.9–1.6% of gestation complicated by HELLP syndrome.
- AFLP and HELLP syndrome are coexistent in approximately 50% of patients. Hypoglycemia is a valued finding in the differential diagnosis with preeclampsia and HELLP syndrome.

REFERENCES

1. Joshi D, James A, Quaglia A, Westbrook RH, Heneghan MA. Liver disease in pregnancy. Lancet. 2010;375(9714):594-605.
2. Shao Z, Al Tibi M, Wakim-Fleming J. Update on viral hepatitis in pregnancy. Clevel Clin J Med. 2017;84(3):202-6.
3. American College of Obstetricians and Gynecologists. ACOG practice bulletin No. 86: Viral hepatitis in pregnancy. Obstet Gynecol. 2007;110:941-56.
4. World Health Organization. (2022). Hepatitis A. [online] Available from www.who.int/mediacentre/factsheets/fs328/en/. [Last accessed April, 2023].
5. US Centers for Disease Control and Prevention (CDC). (2013). Viral Hepatitis Surveillance—United States, 2013. [online] Available from https://www.cdc.gov/hepatitis/statistics/2013surveillance/pdfs/2013hepsurveillancerpt.pdf. [Last accessed April, 2023].
6. Society for Maternal-Fetal Medicine (SMFM); Dionne-Odom J, Tita ATN, Silverman NS. #38: Hepatitis B in pregnancy screening, treatment and prevention of vertical transmission. Am J Obstet Gynecol. 2016;214:6-14.
7. Zou H, Chen Y, Duan Z, Zhang H, Pan C. Virologic factors associated with failure to passive-active immune-prophylaxis in infants born to HBsAg positive mothers. J Viral Hepat. 2012;19:e18-25.
8. Tran TT, Ahn J, Reau NS. ACG Clinical Guideline: Liver Disease and Pregnancy. Am J Gastroenterol. 2016;111:176-94.
9. Schillie S, Wester C, Osborne M, Wesolowski L, Ryerson AB. CDC Recommendations for Hepatitis C Screening Among Adults—United States, 2020. MMWR Recomm Rep. 2020;69(2):1-17.
10. Williamson C, Geenes V. intrahepatic cholestasis of pregnancy. Obstet Gynecol. 2014;124(1);120-33.
11. Wood AM, Livingston EG, Hughes BL, Kuller JA. Intrahepatic cholestasis of pregnancy; a review of diagnosis and management. Obstet Gynecol Surv. 2018;73(2);103-9.
12. Kenyon AP, Tribe RM, Nelson-Piercy C, Girling JC, Williamson C, Seed PT, et al. Pruritus in pregnancy; a study of anatomical distribution and prevalence in relation to the development of obstetric cholestasis. Obstet Med. 2010;3:25-9.
13. Date RS, Kaushal M, Ramesh A. A review of management of gallstone disease and its complications in pregnancy. Am J Surg. 2008;196(4);599-608.
14. Ghumman E, Barry M, Grace PA. Management of gall stone in pregnancy. Br J Surg. 1997;84:1646-50.
15. Kenyon AP, Piercy CN, Girling J, Williamson C, Tribe RM, Shennan AH. Obstetric cholestasis, outcome with active management: a series of 70 cases. BJOG. 2002;109;282-8.
16. Bacq Y, Sapey T, Brechot MC, Pierre F, Fignon A, Dubois F. Intrahepatic cholestasis of pregnancy: a French prospective study. Hepatology. 1997;26:358-64.
17. Reid R, Ivey KJ, Rencoret RH, Storey B. Fetal complications of obstetric cholestasis. Br Med J. 1976;1:870-2.
18. Fisk NM, Storey GN. Fetal outcome in obstetric cholestasis. Br J Obstet Gynaecol. 1988;95:1937-43.
19. Joshi D, James A, Quaglia A, Westbrook RH, Heneghan MA. Liver disease in pregnancy. Lancet. 2010;375(9714):594-605.
20. Rasheed SM, Abdel Monem AM, Abd Ellah AH, Abdel Fattah MS. Prognosis and determinants of pregnancy outcome among patients with post hepatitis liver cirrhosis. Int J Gynaecol Obstet. 2013;121;247-51.
21. Aggarwal N, Negi N, Aggarwal A, Bodh V, Dhiman RK. Pregnancy with portal hypertension. J Clin Exp Hepatol. 2014;4(2);163-71.
22. Chaudhuri K, Tan EK, Biswas A. Successful pregnancy in a woman with liver cirrhosis complicated by recurrent variceal bleeding. J Obstet Gynaecol. 2012;32:490-1.
23. Almashhrawl AA, Ahmed KT, Rahman RN, Hammoud GM, Ibdah JA. Liver diseases in pregnancy: Diseases not unique to pregnancy. World J Gastroenterol. 2013;19;7630-8.

24. Ilhan M, Ilhan G, Gok AFK. The course and outcomes of complicated gallstone disease in pregnancy: Experience of a tertiary center. Turk J Obstet Gynecol. 2016;13(4): 178-82.
25. Liu J, Ghaziani TT, Wolf JL. Acute fatty liver disease of pregnancy: updates in pathogenesis, diagnosis and management. Am. J Gastroenterol. 2017;112(6):838-46.
26. Lamprecht A, Morton A, Laurie J, Lee W. Acute fatty liver of pregnancy and concomitant medical conditions: A review of cases at a quaternary obstetric hospital. Obstet Med. 2018;11(4):178-81.
27. Bacak SJ, Thornburg LL. Liver failure in pregnancy. Crit Care Clin. 2016;32(1): 61-72.
28. Knight M, Nelson-Piercy C, Kurinczuk JJ, Spark P, Brocklehurst P; UK Obstetric Surveillance System. A prospective national study of acute fatty liver of pregnancy in the UK. Gut. 2008;57(7):951-6.
29. Sibai BM. Imitators of severe preeclampsia. Obstet Gynecol. 2007;109(4):956-66.
30. Deshpande NA, James NT, Kucirka LM, Boyarsky BJ, Garonzik-Wang JM, Cameron AM, et al. Pregnancy outcomes of liver transplant recipients: a systemic review and meta-analysis. Liver Transpl. 2012;18(6):621-9.
31. Scantleburry V, Gordon R, Tzakis A, Koneru B, Bowman J, Mazzaferro V, et al. Childbearing after liver transplantation. Transplantation. 1990;49(2):317-21.
32. Goodwin TM. Hyperemesis gravidarum. Obstet Gynecol Clin North Am. 2008;35(3): 401-17.
33. Bailit JL. Hyperemesis gravidarum: Epidemiologic findings from a large cohort. Am J Obstet Gynecol. 2005;193(3):811-4.
34. Saphier CJ, Repke JT. Hemolysis, elevated liver enzymes, and low platelets (HELLP) syndrome: a review of diagnosis and management. Semin Perinatol. 1998; 22:118-33.

Renal Disorders in Pregnancy

Manoj Chellani

INTRODUCTION

Approximately 3% of pregnant women are affected by the renal disease in developed countries. The prevalence of renal disease in pregnancy is predicted to rise in the future due to increasing maternal age and obesity. Although it is not a barrier to reproduction in most women.[1]

The risk of adverse pregnancy outcomes is increased in women and it is associated with including preeclampsia, loss of maternal renal function, and fetal growth restriction. Moreover, chronic kidney disease (CKD) impacts communication, decision-making, and the surveillance and management of women before, during, and after pregnancy. Therefore, planning of pregnancy is crucial to optimize maternal management and proper understanding of the risks. In this chapter, main physiologic changes and renal disorders in pregnancy were discussed.

PHYSIOLOGIC CHANGES IN PREGNANCY

The physiologic changes in pregnancy are given as **Table 1**.

Glomerular Filtration Rate

Anatomic changes begin in the first trimester of pregnancy and can persist up to 16 weeks postpartum. The length of the kidney increases by 1–1.5 cm and volume up by 30%.[2]

TABLE 1: Physiologic changes in pregnancy.

Increased	Decreased
• Blood volume	• Systemic vascular resistance
• Cardiac output	
• Levels of nitric oxide and relaxin	• Systemic blood pressure
• Relative resistance to vasoconstrictors	• Serum creatinine
	• Th2
• Glomerular filtration rate (GFR) by 50%	• Tregs
	• GFR
• Urine protein excretion	
• T helper type 2 (Th2) phenotype	
• Circulation of regulatory T cell (Treg)	

The dilatation of the renal calyces, pelvis, uterus, and reduced ureteral peristaltic activity are the main changes in pregnancy. These changes increase about ~40–50% in glomerular filtration rate (GFR), which peaks in the first trimester and were decrease by 15–20% in late third trimester.[3,4] The increased GFR leads to a decrease the serum creatinine and urea together with an increase in protein excretion.[5] The normal serum creatinine in pregnancy is in the 0.4–0.6 mg/dL range.

Blood Pressure

Increased GFR is caused by cardiac output, an increase in renal blood flow, and a decrease in systemic blood pressure usually reaching a nadir by 20 weeks gestation. It may be due to

TABLE 2: Hemodynamics index during normal uncomplicated pregnancy.

	Blood pressure		GFR	RPF
	Systolic	Diastolic		
First trimester (1–12 weeks)	111.5	65.2	+37%	+42%
Second trimester (13–25 weeks)	110.0	64.0	+38.4%	+29.4%
Third trimester (26–36 weeks)	115.0	69.0	+39.5%	10.4%

(GFR: glomerular filtration rate; RPF: renal plasma flow)

vasodilatation and plasma volume increase caused by several signaling molecules that decrease kidney excretion of sodium. There are elevated levels of vasodilators, such as relaxin and nitric oxide, and relative resistance to vasoconstrictors, such as angiotensin. **Table 2** summarized the study data on systolic and diastolic blood pressure in a normal uncomplicated pregnancy.[6]

PHYSIOLOGICAL HYDRONEPHROSIS

Hydronephrosis takes place in 43–100% of the pregnancy, and it is more prevalent with the advancing trimester.[7] The highest incidence of hydronephrosis is touched at 28 weeks, with a 63% overall incidence of hydronephrosis. The distended collecting system can hold 200–300 mL of urine, leading to urinary stasis and a 40% increased possibility for pyelonephritis in pregnant women with asymptomatic bacteriuria versus nonpregnant women. Physiologic hydronephrosis may arise due to the combination of progesterone and mechanical compression by the enlarging uterus.[8]

PROTEINURIA

Proteinuria is one of the vital features of preeclampsia, a common and potentially severe complication of pregnancy. Proteinuria in pregnancy can also indicate primary kidney disease or kidney disease secondary to systemic disorders, such as diabetes mellitus or primary hypertension. Proteinuria is a key sign of kidney impairment and a risk element for kidney disease development. Urinary protein excretion increases in normal pregnancy from 60–90 mg/d to 180–250 mg/d, as measured by a 24-hour urine collection. Thus, the threshold of abnormal protein excretion for the diagnosis of preeclampsia is >300 mg/24 hours or >2 + by dipstick testing according to the American College of Obstetricians and Gynecologists guidelines.[9,10] The increase in proteinuria has been attributed to hyperfiltration, but it may also be due to changes in glomerular permeability. Some studies have demonstrated an increase in tubular proteinuria, reflected as an increase in urinary retinol-binding protein, as opposed to an increase in albuminuria, which would reflect a glomerular source.[11]

INNATE AND ADAPTIVE IMMUNITY

There are several changes in the function of the innate and adaptive immune systems in pregnancy that may have important impacts on the behavior of autoimmune diseases, a common cause of reduced kidney function in young women. Normal pregnancy is characterized by a shift from a T helper type 1 (Th1) (cell-mediated immunity) to a T helper type 2 (Th2) (humoral-mediated immunity) phenotype, which is important for tolerance to fetal antigens, trophoblast invasion, and placental formation. In addition, the number of regulatory T cells (Tregs), which promote immune tolerance, is increased in normal pregnancy, further contributing to establishing fetal tolerance. In autoimmune diseases, such as systemic lupus erythematosus (SLE), alterations in the number and function of Tregs may correlate with an increased risk for pregnancy complications, such as preeclampsia and poor fetal and maternal outcomes.[12]

PATHOGENESIS OF PREGNANCY-RELATED DISORDERS

In the pregnant population with lupus, the most frequent maternal complications include relapse of lupus (25.6%), hypertension (16.3%), lupus nephritis (16.1%), and preeclampsia (7.6%).[13] Patients with established lupus nephritis had a higher risk of hypertension and premature birth. Antiphospholipid antibodies were associated with arterial hypertension, premature delivery, and abortion.[14]

HYPERTENSIVE DISORDERS OF PREGNANCY

Hypertensive disorders of pregnancy are common, occurring in 6–8% of pregnancies. The differential diagnosis of hypertensive events during pregnancy includes chronic hypertension, gestational hypertension, or preeclampsia.

Chronic Hypertension

Chronic hypertension is considered when patients' blood pressure is ≥140/90 mm Hg before 20 weeks of pregnancy or any known history of hypertension before the pregnancy.

Gestational Hypertension

A few hypertensive patients with unidentified histories of hypertension before the pregnancy may be existing with normal blood pressures in the first and second trimesters due to the usual and physiologic drop in blood pressure seen during this time, thus hiding the diagnosis of preexisting hypertension. This may lead to the erroneous assumption that the finding of elevated blood pressure later during pregnancy is related to gestational hypertension.

The exact diagnosis eventually is confirmed throughout the postpartum period, as blood pressure should normalize in those with true gestational hypertension. Gestational hypertension is more common during the second trimester of pregnancy in patients with no prior history of preexisting hypertension, with a prevalence of 6-7%. In a meta-analysis of the effects of antihypertensives on fetal growth, a significant association between mean arterial pressure and fetal weight was identified, with a 10 mm Hg drop in mean arterial pressure associated with a 176 g decline in fetal birth weight. Therefore, proper timely management of hypertension is important as for the national and international guideline.[15]

Guidelines

Treatment guidelines in pregnancy something differ across obstetric societies and countries, the American, UK, and Canadian guidelines[16-18] are as follows:
- The American guidelines recommend the initial antihypertensive therapy in patients with gestational hypertension or preeclampsia with a persistent blood pressure of ≥160/110 mm Hg, and delivery is recommended for these women at 37 weeks or later.

- The National Institute for Health and Care Excellence (NICE) guidelines in the United Kingdom, recommends initiation of treatment at systolic blood pressures ≥150 mm Hg and/or diastolic blood pressures ≥100 mm Hg.
- Canadian guidelines recommend initiating treatment at a blood pressure ≥140/90 mm Hg.

■ PREECLAMPSIA

Preeclampsia is recognized as high blood pressure ≥140/90 mm Hg in an earlier normal hypertensive woman, measured on two different times, at least 4 hours apart, after 20 weeks of gestation, in the occurrence of proteinuria ≥300 mg/d, or a protein/creatinine ratio ≥0.3 g/g. The etiology of preeclampsia is unknown but it is thought to be due to endothelial damage. Routine antenatal care includes screening for preeclampsia through regular blood pressure measurements and urinalysis to detect proteinuria. A diagnosis of preeclampsia also can be made in the absence of proteinuria in the presence of clinical features of severity. **Table 3** summarized the clinical features of risk factors, symptoms, and signs of preeclampsia.[19] The use of spot urine protein-creatinine ratio (UPCR) has grown favor in the diagnosis of preeclampsia, which is usually characterized by proteinuria (UCPR >0.3 g/g). The UPCR is a faster test that has an acceptable sensitivity and specificity.[4]

Preeclampsia Management

Preeclampsia is associated with increased risks of fetal growth restriction and placental abruption. In the past two decades, the heterogeneity of preeclampsia with respect to fundamental mechanisms and ensuing clinical phenotypes has been progressively documented. Main improvements in the pathophysiology of preeclampsia have confirmed that attributed compromised angiogenesis in preeclampsia to an imbalance between proangiogenic and antiangiogenic factors favoring the latter. However, angiogenic abnormalities seem to be informative for severe and early (<34 weeks of gestation) forms of preeclampsia, but not for late disease (≥34 weeks of gestation). Women with preeclampsia have higher circulating levels of soluble fms-like tyrosine kinase 1 (sFlt-1), which binds and antagonizes angiogenic placental growth factor (PlGF) and vascular endothelial

TABLE 3: Preeclampsia: common risk factors, symptoms, and signs.

Common risk factors	Symptoms	Signs
• Age >40 years • Obesity • Previous personal history or family history of preeclampsia • Primiparity • Long inter-birth interval • Multiple pregnancies • Preexisting hypertension • Chronic kidney disease • Diabetes/gestational diabetes • Connective tissue disorders and the presence of antiphospholipid antibodies	• Headache • Visual disturbances including flashing lights • Epigastric/right upper quadrant pain • Nausea and vomiting • Rapidly increasing/severe swelling of face, hands, and lower limbs	• Hypertension • Proteinuria (new onset) • Epigastric/right upper quadrant tenderness • Papilledema • Clonus (>3 beats is significant) • Convulsions/mental disorientation • Biochemical parameters: • Elevated serum transaminases • Thrombocytopenia • Hemolysis • Raised creatinine • Raised uric acid

growth factor (VEGF). In women without CKD, several studies have defined predictive values of sFlt:PlGF ratio or PlGF alone to guide clinical management.[4]

The only available screening method that has a considerable net advantage is serial blood pressure measurements throughout pregnancy. Patients with a moderate or high risk of preeclampsia can benefit with is low-dose aspirin when prescribed during the late first trimester; patients with a history of preeclampsia and preterm delivery at <34 weeks; and those with a history of preeclampsia in two or more pregnancies.

ACUTE KIDNEY INJURY IN PREGNANCY

Pregnancy-related acute kidney injury (AKI) in young women worldwide is an important cause of maternal and fetal morbidity and mortality. AKI etiology varies geographically and according to the availability of health resources. In the past, the main cause of AKI during pregnancy in developing countries is severe sepsis from septic abortions and hyperemesis gravidarum in the first trimester. Other causes of AKI include hypertensive disorders of pregnancy and hemorrhage and acute liver disease in second and third trimesters.[20,21] In developed countries, causes of AKI also include hypertensive disorders of pregnancy and sepsis, as well as thrombotic microangiopathy, heart failure, acute fatty liver, and postpartum hemorrhage.[21] Nowadays, preeclampsia is leading cause of AKI mainly in developed countries, while in developing countries where abortion is illegal, septic abortion is a frequent cause of AKI.[1,22,23]

Rates of pregnancy-related AKI overall have decreased in the last several decades, most likely due to improved prenatal care and a decrease in septic abortions. AKI requiring dialysis in pregnancy or postpartum is even less common, occurring in 1 per 10,000 pregnant women, but it is associated with increased mortality. AKI can be categorized as prerenal, intrinsic, or postrenal. Prerenal conditions are the most common causes of AKI and usually result from inadequate perfusion of the kidneys. The obstetric complications of AKI include hemorrhage from the placenta previa, abruption placenta, and uterine atony **(Box 1)**. AKI from renal hypoperfusion is usually reversible within 24–36 hours with volume replacement and correction of the underlying cause. Without prompt treatment, acute tubular necrosis (ATN) may develop. Most of the deaths from AKI in pregnancy are due to the following disease rather than renal failure itself.[24]

BOX 1: Reasons of AKI in pregnancy.
- Preeclampsia-eclampsia
- HELLP syndrome
- Severe peripartum hemorrhage
- Placental abruption
- Disseminated intravascular coagulation secondary to a prolonged fetal demise
- Uterine atony
- Uterine lacerations and perforations
- Uterine dehiscence of cesarean scar
- Septic shock
- Chorioamnionitis
- Septic abortion
- Puerperal sepsis
- Volume depletion
- Hyperemesis gravidarum
- Severe vomiting from pyelonephritis
- Obstruction of gravid uterus
- Hydramnios
- Multiple gestations
- Idiopathic postpartum renal failure
- Amniotic fluid embolism
- Acute fatty liver of pregnancy
- Hemolysis, elevated liver enzymes, and low platelets

(AKI: acute kidney injury; HELLP: hemolysis, elevated liver enzymes, and low platelet count)

Pregnant women may develop AKI from multiple causes beyond the pregnancy-related disorders mentioned above. Renal complications can potentially be generated from interventions such as renal support therapy and infections associated with an intravascular device, among others. Hypertensive disorders during pregnancy by themselves can be associated with a risk of preterm delivery and consequently a decrease in nephron mass, making this a risk factor for developing CKD in adulthood.[25-27] Although current evidence is limited, but some studies suggest that episodes of AKI are associated with an increased risk of CKD and the development of preeclampsia in the mother.[28]

ACUTE CORTICAL NECROSIS

The most serious complication of acute renal failure (ARF) is bilateral renal cortical necrosis (BRCN). The condition occurs when the death of renal cortical tissue with sparing of the medulla. However, it is unclear but researcher suggested that it may be due to endothelial damage done by endotoxin followed by the formation of thrombi.[29]

The underestimation of the occurrence of BRCN because of patchy cortical necrosis with partial or nearly complete recovery or renal function may be ignored if a patient survives and suitable investigations are not carried. Abruption placenta is the most common pregnancy complication related with BRCN, whereas the occurrence is comparatively low in patients with severe preeclampsia. BRCN should be strongly assumed if ARF develops before 30 weeks of gestation and is related with prolonged anuria or oliguria (of >10 days duration). Anuria or oliguria is the rule, and urine is usually blood-stained. Renal biopsy or selective arteriography can be used to confirm the diagnosis and distinguish between extensive and patchy cortical necrosis.[30]

CHRONIC RENAL DISEASE IN PREGNANCY

Chronic renal failure is defined as a decrease in renal mass and loss of renal reserve following renal injury. The common chronic renal conditions include diabetic nephropathy, lupus nephritis, and solid organ transplantation. Chronic renal failure has multiple etiologies; SLE, diabetes, and hypertension have replaced glomerulonephritis (nephrotic syndrome, idiopathic membranous nephropathy, and focal segmental glomerulosclerosis) as a major etiology. Renal insufficiency is categorized as mild, moderate, or severe.[31,32]

- *Mild renal disease:* Patient's serum creatinine level of 1.4 mg/dL or less, or 125 µmol/L or less, and no hypertension.
- *Moderate renal insufficiency:* Patients have a serum creatinine level of 1.5–2.5 mg/dL, or 125–250 µmol/L.
- *Severe renal disease:* Patients have a creatinine level of 2.5 mg/dL or more, or 250 µmol/L or more.

Maternal and perinatal outcomes are usually not affected with mild renal insufficiency. Similarly, the effects of pregnancy do not deteriorate renal function when mildly diminished. Whereas moderate and severe CKD cause increased fetal growth restriction and preterm deliveries.[33,34]

The prevalence of CKD increases with age. Thus, the overall prevalence of CKD among pregnant women is low. However, CKD increases the risk of adverse maternal and fetal outcomes in proportion to the stage and severity of the disease. Among pregnant women with CKD, 40% developed preeclampsia, 48% developed anemia, and

56% developed chronic hypertension.[35] Approximately 20% of pregnant women developing preeclampsia before 30 weeks of gestation have previously undiagnosed CKD, especially those with severe proteinuria.[36] CKD stages 3–5 have been estimated to affect one every 750 pregnant women.[36]

The study in England in 1996 defined end-stage renal disease as a serum creatinine level of >6.0 mg/dL, and a change in renal function was defined as a 25% change in the equation 1/serum creatinine, which linearly associates with GFR. Overall, the total rate of decline in renal function was 43%; renal function declined in 11 women during pregnancy and in 16 after delivery.[37]

All pregnant women with CKD should be monitored during gestation by a multidisciplinary team involving specialists in obstetrics, nephrology, urology, fetal medicine, and neonatology, being at risk for pregnancy-related adverse events. The frequency of follow-up must be adapted to the severity of the disease; for example, in CKD stages 3–5, follow-up should be intensified. Follow-up of pregnant women with CKD is basic for the early recognition and treatment of complications, including proteinuria, anemia, coagulation disorders, hypertension, and systemic diseases.

SYSTEMIC LUPUS ERYTHEMATOSUS

Systemic lupus erythematosus affects reproductive-aged women. Women with SLE can *extremely* flare during pregnancy, in particular those who have active disease at beginning of pregnancy or prior history of renal disease. These flares can lead to increased adverse pregnancy outcomes including fetal loss, preeclampsia, preterm birth, and small for gestational aged infants. In addition, women with antiphospholipid antibodies can have thrombosis during pregnancy or higher rates of fetal loss.

Epidemiologic studies estimate the occurrence of SLE is among 45.2–102.9 per 100,000 with an incidence of 2.4–7.2 per 100,000/year.[38,39] The highest incidence of SLE is seen in women, peaking during their reproductive years.[40,41]

The increase in incidence among women may be due to the fact that X chromosome and sex hormones have been related with immune dysregulation. The hazardous gene for SLE has been identified on the X chromosome (e.g., Foxp3, TLR7, IRAK1, and CD40 ligand), and estrogens have effects on B cell maturation, antibody production, Th2 responses, and survival of autoreactive cells.[41]

In the study of 155 patients with lupus who became pregnant, active lupus at the time of conception was associated with renal and hematologic flares. In this cohort, 6.1% of women with the active disease during pregnancy died and 15.9% developed organ failures.[42]

The study recommends that all pregnant women with SLE should continue hydroxychloroquine unless contraindicated. Given the risk of pre-eclampsia, and adding low-dose aspirin at the end of the first trimester is beneficial. Transition women who need ongoing immunosuppression for disease control to an immunosuppressive agent compatible with pregnancy (e.g., tacrolimus, azathioprine, or cyclosporine) and observe for 4–6 months to make certain that the disease is stable prior to conception.

DIABETIC NEPHROPATHY

Diabetic nephropathy is a hurdle that can occur in 4–10% of pregnancies in women with diabetes. The pathology of diabetic nephropathy is glomerulosclerosis, either diffuse or nodular. This disorder typically occurs with heavy proteinuria, azotemia, and hypertension. The exact reason for diabetic nephropathy is unidentified but has been endorsed to glycemic control, hypertension, an increase in GFR, or an increase in protein intake and excretion, all of which are affected by pregnancy.[43]

It is unclear whether diabetic nephropathy is accelerated by pregnancy. A few studies have shown that pregnancy has an adverse effect on diabetic nephropathy, increasing proteinuria, and creatinine clearance.[44,45] Other studies have not observed any progression or development of nephropathy in women with diabetes.[46-50]

Women with diabetic nephropathy are at increased risk for adverse maternal and fetal growth impairment, especially preterm delivery, intrauterine growth restriction (IUGR), preeclampsia, and hypertensive complications. The rates of preterm delivery at <34 weeks of gestation range from 16 to 31%,[45,46] and the rates of IUGR range from 9 to 22%.[48-53] In addition, the rate of preeclampsia may be as high as 50%. Approximately 10–15% of women with diabetes are affected by pregnancy-induced hypertension.[45,53]

Clinical practice guidelines on pregnancy and renal disease in the United Kingdom recommended that women with diabetic nephropathy have the optimization of blood glucose, blood pressure, and proteinuria prior to conception. If the woman attempting to conceive with diabetic nephropathy she should continue angiotensin-converting enzyme inhibitors until conception, with regular pregnancy testing.[54] The schedule of care, investigation, and supervision of women with diabetic nephropathy should be untaken as for the national guidelines for diabetes in pregnancy, in addition to dedicated monitoring of renal disease in pregnancy.

■ GLOMERULONEPHRITIS

Acute glomerulonephritis (the acute nephritic syndrome) is characterized by the abrupt appearance of red blood cells and red blood cell casts in the urine. Renal function is usually impaired, with sodium and water retention leading to edema and hypertension. The blood urea nitrogen (BUN) and creatinine levels rise and creatinine clearance declines. Proteinuria is common but is normally less than 3.5 g per 24 hours. Renal diseases presenting as acute glomerulonephritis include post-streptococcal glomerulonephritis, lupus glomerulonephritis, membrane proliferative glomerulonephritis, and Goodpasture syndrome. Laboratory investigations may help to distinguish the different causes and should include urine microscopy, creatinine clearance, 24-hour urinary protein collection, serum immunoglobulin A (IgA) and complement determinations, streptozyme assay and antistreptolysin O titers, and evaluation of antinuclear antibody.[55] Management problems include control of hypertension, electrolyte balance, and edema. Uremia may not respond to conservative measures and may require renal dialysis.[24]

■ REFERENCES

1. Piccoli GB, Zakharova E, Attini R, Hernandez MI, Covella B, Alrukhaimi M, et al. Acute kidney injury in pregnancy: the need for higher awareness. A pragmatic review focused on what could be improved in the prevention and care of pregnancy-related AKI, in the year dedicated to women and kidney diseases. J Clin Med. 2018;7:724-35.
2. Maynard SE, Karumanchi SA, Thadhani R. Hypertension and kidney disease in pregnancy. In: Skorecki K, Chertow GM, Marsden PA, Taal MW, Yu ASL (Eds). Brenner and Rector's The Kidney, 10th edition. Philadelphia, PA: Elsevier; 2016. pp. 1610-63.

3. Linheimer MD, Katz AI. Renal physiology and disease in pregnancy. In: Seldin DW, Giebisch G (Eds). The Kidney: Physiology and Pathophysiology, 3rd edition. Philadelphia: Lippincott Williams & Wilkins; 2000.
4. Gonzalez Suarez ML, Kattah A, Grande JP, Garovic V. Renal disorders in pregnancy: core curriculum 2019. Am J Kidney Dis. 2019;73:119-30.
5. Dissanayake VH, Morgan L, Broughton Pipkin F, Vathanan V, Premaratne S, Jayasekara RW, et al. The urine protein heat coagulation test—a useful screening test for proteinuria in pregnancy in developing countries: a method validation study. BJOG. 2004;111:491-4.
6. Mcdonald-Wallis C, Silverwood RJ, Fraser A, Nelson SM, Tilling K, Lawlor DA, et al. Gestational-age-specific reference ranges for blood pressure in pregnancy: findings from a prospective cohort. J Hypertens. 2015;33:96-105.
7. Faundes A, Bricola-Filho M, Pinto e Silva JL. Dilatation of the urinary tract during pregnancy: proposal of a curve of maximal caliceal diameter by gestational age. Am J Obstet Gynecol. 1998;178(5):1082-6.
8. Cietak KA, Newton JR. Serial quantitative maternal nephrosonography in pregnancy. Br J Radiol. 1985;58(689):405-13.
9. ACOG Practice Bulletin No. 202: Gestational Hypertension and Preeclampsia. Obstet Gynecol. 2019;133:1.
10. Thornton CE, Makris A, Ogle RF, Tooher JM, Hennessy A. Role of proteinuria in defining pre-eclampsia: clinical outcomes for women and babies. Clin Exp Pharmacol Physiol. 2010;37:466-70.
11. Osman O, Maynard S. Proteinuria in pregnancy-Review. Front Womens Healt. 2019;(4):1-5.
12. Piccinni MP, Lombardelli L, Logiodice F, Kullolli O, Parronchi P, Romagnani S. How pregnancy can affect autoimmune diseases progression? Clin Mol Allergy. 2016;14:11.
13. Cabarcas-Barbosa O, Capalbo O, Ferrero-Fernández A, Musso CG. Kidney–placenta crosstalk in health and disease. Clin Kidney J. 2022;15(7):1284-9.
14. Clausen P, Ekbom P, Damm P, Feldt-Rasmussen U, Nielsen B, Mathiesen ER, et al. Signs of maternal vascular dysfunction precede preeclampsia in women with type 1 diabetes. J Diabetes Complications. 2007;21:288-93.
15. Oliverio AL, Bramham K, Hladunewich MA. Pregnancy and CKD: Advances in Care and the Legacy of Dr Susan Hou. Am J Kidney Dis. 2021;78(6):865-75.
16. American College of Obstetricians and Gynecologists' Committee on Practice Bulletins—Obstetrics. ACOG Practice Bulletin No. 203: Chronic hypertension in pregnancy. Obstet Gynecol. 2019;133(1):e26-50.
17. National Institute for Health and Care Excellence. (2019). Hypertension in pregnancy: diagnosis and management. [online] Available from www.nice.org.uk/guidance/ng133. [Last accessed April, 2023].
18. Butalia S, Audibert F, Côté AM, Firoz T, Logan AG, Magee LA, et al. Hypertension Canada's 2018 guidelines for the management of hypertension in pregnancy. Can J Cardiol. 2018;34(5):526-31.
19. Palma-Reis I, Vais A, Nelson-Piercy C, Banerjee A. Renal disease and hypertension in pregnancy. Clin Med (Lond). 2013;13(1):57-62.
20. Rao S, Jim B. Acute kidney injury in pregnancy: the changing landscape for the 21st century. Kidney Int Rep. 2018;3:247-57.
21. Jim B, Garovic VD. Acute kidney injury in pregnancy. Semin Nephrol. 2017;37:378-85.
22. Prakash J, Pant P, Prakash S, Sivasankar M, Vohra R, Doley PK, et al. Changing picture of acute kidney injury in pregnancy: study of 259 cases over a period of 33 years. Indian J Nephrol. 2016;26:262-7.
23. Mahesh E, Puri S, Varma V, Madhyastha PR, Bande S, Gurudev KC. Pregnancy-related acute kidney injury: an analysis of 165 cases. Indian J Nephrol. 2017;27:113-7.
24. Hnat M, Sibai B. (2008). Renal Disease and Pregnancy. [online] Available from https://www.glowm.com/section-view/heading/Renal%20Disease%20and%20Pregnancy/item/157#. [Last accessed April, 2023].

25. Low Birth Weight and Nephron Number Working Group. The impact of kidney development on the life course: a consensus document for action. Nephron. 2017;136:3-49.
26. Luyckx VA, Bertram JF, Brenner BM, Fall C, Hoy WE, Ozanne SE, et al. Effect of fetal and child health on kidney development and long-term risk of hypertension and kidney disease. Lancet. 2013;382:273-83.
27. Luyckx VA, Brenner BM. Birth weight, malnutrition and kidney-associated outcomes—a global concern. Nat Rev Nephrol. 2015;11:135-49.
28. Tangren JS, Powe CE, Ankers E, Ecker J, Bramham K, Hladunewich MA, et al. Pregnancy outcomes after clinical recovery from AKI. J Am Soc Nephrol. 2017;28:1566-74.
29. Lindheimer MD, Katz Al, Ganeval D. Acute renal failure in pregnancy. In: Brenner BM, Lazara JM (Eds). Acute Renal Failure. Philadelphia: WB Saunders; 1983. pp. 510.
30. Kleinknecht D, Grünfeld JP, Gomez PC, Moreau JF, Garcia-Torres R. Diagnostic procedures and long-term prognosis in bilateral renal cortical necrosis. Kidney Int. 1973;4:390-400.
31. Davison JM, Lindheimer MD. Renal disorders. In: Davison JM (Ed). Maternal-Fetal Medicine. Philadelphia: WB Saunders; 1999.
32. Jones DC. Pregnancy complicated by chronic renal disease. Clin Perinatol. 1997;24:483-96.
33. Ramin SM, Vidaeff AC, Yeomans ER, Gilstrap LC 3rd. Chronic renal disease in pregnancy. Obstet Gynecol. 2006;108:1531-9.
34. Doi K, Rabb H. Impact of acute kidney injury on distant organ function: recent findings and potential therapeutic targets. Kidney Int. 2016;89:555-64.
35. Trevisan G, Ramos JGL, Martins-Costa S, Guardão Barros EJ. Pregnancy in patients with chronic renal insufficiency at Hospital de Clínicas of Porto Alegre, Brazil. Ren Fail. 2004;26:29-34.
36. Williams D, Davison J. Chronic kidney disease in pregnancy. BMJ. 2008;336(7637):211-5.
37. Jones DC, Hayslett JP. Outcome of pregnancy in women with moderate or severe renal insufficiency. N Engl J Med. 1996;335:226-32.
38. Gergianaki I, Bortoluzzi A, Bertsias G. Update on the epidemiology, risk factors, and disease outcomes of systemic lupus erythematosus. Best Pract Res Clin Rheumatol. 2018;32(2):188-205.
39. Stojan G, Petri M. Epidemiology of systemic lupus erythematosus: an update. Curr Opin Rheumatol. 2018;30(2):144-50.
40. Gaudreau MC, Johnson BM, Gudi R, Al-Gadban MM, Vasu C. Gender bias in lupus: does immune response initiated in the gut mucosa have a role? Clin Exp Immunol. 2015;180(3):393-407.
41. Tedeschi SK, Bermas B, Costenbader KH. Sexual disparities in the incidence and course of SLE and RA. Clin Immunol. 2013;149(2):211-8.
42. Yang H, Liu H, Xu D, Zhao L, Wang Q, Leng X, et al. Pregnancy-related systemic lupus erythematosus: clinical features, outcome and risk factors of disease flares–a case control study. PLoS One. 2014;9(8):e104375.
43. Rosenn BM, Miodovnik M. Medical complications of diabetes mellitus in pregnancy. Clin Obstet Gynecol. 2000;43:17-31.
44. Biesenbach G, Stoger H, Zazgornik J. Influence of pregnancy on progression of diabetic nephropathy and subsequent requirement of renal replacement therapy in female type I diabetic patients with impaired renal function. Nephrol Dial Transplant. 1992;7:105-9.
45. Gordon M, Landon MB, Samuels P, Hissrich S, Gabbe SG. Perinatal outcome and long-term follow-up associated with modern management of diabetic nephropathy. Obstet Gynecol. 1996;87:401-9.
46. Kitzmiller JL, Brown ER, Phillippe M, Stark AR, Acker D, Kaldany A. et al. Diabetic nephropathy and perinatal outcome. Am J Obstet Gynecol. 1981;141:741-51.
47. Grenfell A, Brudenell JM, Doddridge MC, Watkins PJ. Pregnancy in diabetic women who have proteinuria. Q J Med. 1986;59:379-86.

48. Kimmerle R, Zass RP, Cupisti S, Somville T, Bender R, Pawlowski B, et al. Pregnancies in women with diabetic nephropathy: Long-term outcome for mother and child. Diabetologia. 1995;38:227-35.
49. Mackie A, Doddridge MC, Gamsu HR, Brudenell JM, Nicolaides KH, Drury PL. Outcome of pregnancy in patients with insulin-dependent diabetes mellitus and nephropathy with moderate renal impairment. Diabetes Med. 1996;13: 90-6.
50. Hemachandra A, Lloyd CE, Ellis D, Orchard TJ. The influence of pregnancy on IDDM complications. Diabetes Care. 1995; 18:950-4.
51. Reece EA, Coustan DR, Hayslett JP, Holford T, Coulehan J, O'Connor TZ. et al. Diabetic nephropathy: Pregnancy performance and fetomaternal outcome. Am J Obstet Gynecol. 1998;159:56-66.
52. Jovanovic R, Jovanovic L. Obstetric management when normoglycemia is maintained in diabetic pregnant women with vascular compromise. Am J Obstet Gynecol. 1984;149:617-23.
53. Reece E, Leguizamon G, Homko C. Stringent control in diabetic nephropathy associated with optimization of pregnancy outcomes. J Matern Fetal Med. 1998;7:213-6.
54. Wiles K, Chappell L, Clark K, Elman L, Hall M, Lightstone L, et al. Clinical practice guideline on pregnancy and renal disease. BMC Nephrol. 2019;20:401.
55. Couser WG. Glomerular disorders. In Wyngaarden JB, Smith LH (Eds). Textbook of Medicine, 17th edition. Philadelphia: WB Saunders; 1985. pp. 578.

10

Epilepsy in Pregnancy

Rajasri G Yaliwal, Neelamma Patil, Sangamesh B Bhagavati

■ INTRODUCTION

Epilepsy is a commonly encountered neurological disease. It affects 1% of the population in India. The prevalence of epilepsy at any point of time has said to be 6.38 per 1,000 persons.[1] It is said that the prevalence is underestimated as a lot of people in the rural areas go under diagnosed. It is one of the oldest described disorders with scripts dated back to 4,000 BC.[2] Women with epilepsy (WWE) face many issues during the reproductive age. They would require advice on contraception, prepregnancy counseling, special care during pregnancy, and during the postpartum period. Many misconceptions regarding the epilepsy existed in the past, including equating it to insanity. This would prevent a woman from marriage according to the Hindu Marriage act of 1955. However, The Marriage Law Amendment Act of 1999 recognized the difference between insanity and epilepsy and hence WWE regained their right to marry. The Act also said that epilepsy was neither a reason to divorce or annul a marriage.

■ DEFINITION OF EPILEPSY

The definition of epilepsy has undergone changes. The "International League Against Epilepsy (ILAE)" considers epilepsy to be a brain disease which fulfils any one of the criteria: (1) at least two unprovoked (or reflex) seizures occurring >24 hours apart; (2) one unprovoked (or reflex) seizure and a probability of further seizures similar to the general recurrence risk (at least 60%) after two unprovoked seizures, occurring over the next 10 years; and (3) diagnosis of an epilepsy syndrome.[3]

■ CLASSIFICATION OF EPILEPSY

The classification of types of epilepsy has also undergone changes. According to the ILAE 2017 guidelines several categories have been made which are depicted in **Figure 1**.[4]

■ ANTIEPILEPTIC DRUGS

Women with epilepsy would require special attention during reproductive years and during the postpartum period as many of the antiepileptic drugs (AEDs) interact with oral contraceptives. She would require to make necessary choices in the contraceptive method that she would have to adopt. Many women would be on AEDs prior to conception. It is the duty of the treating doctor to bring about awareness of the adverse effects that the drugs could have on contraception and pregnancy. The WWE may need to change the AED that she is on so that it would not react to contraceptive drugs and minimize the chance of congenital malformations in the fetus if planning for pregnancy.

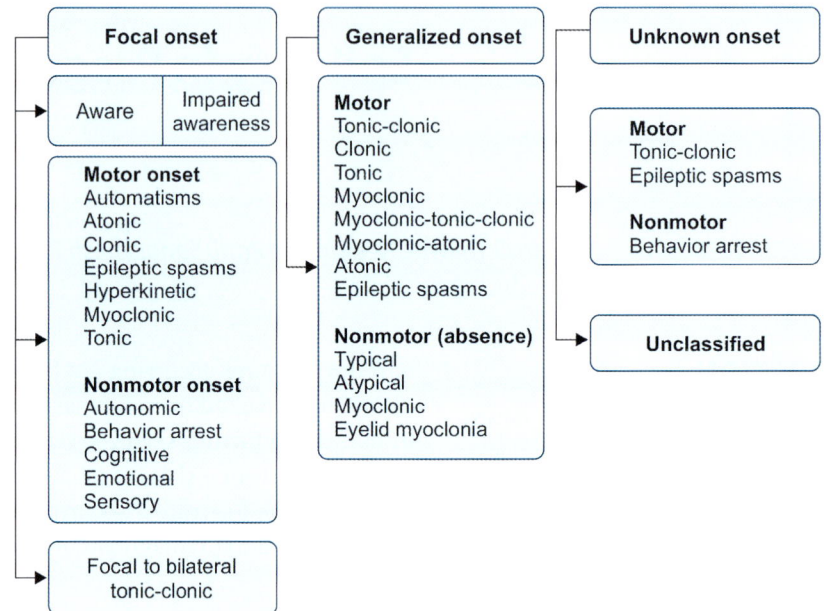

Fig. 1: The International League Against Epilepsy (ILAE) 2017 classification of seizure types expanded version.

Classification of Antiepileptic Drugs

The AEDs are classified as per the time that they were discovered.
- *First-generation AED:* These drugs were developed during the early 1900s. These are phenobarbital, phenytoin, primidone, and ethosuximide.
- *Second-generation AED:* These drugs were developed after the 1990 and have fewer drug interactions and adverse effects. They are vigabatrin, zonisamide, lamotrigine, gabapentin, topiramate, fosphenytoin, tiagabine, oxcarbamazepine, levetiracetam, and pregabalin.
- *Third-generation AED:* Lacosamide, rufinamide, eslicarbazepine, perampanel, and brivaracetam.[5]

Commonly used Antiepileptic Drugs

Phenytoin
- *Mechanism of action:* This drug acts by modulating of voltage-dependent ion channels, Na^+, Ca^{2+}, and K^+
- $t\frac{1}{2}$: 6–60 hours
- Has strong protein-binding action, i.e., 87–93%, hence efficacy could be low in conditions where serum albumin is low
- *Dosage:* 200–400 mg/day
- Administered one to two times a day
- Has interaction with estrogen-containing oral contraceptive pills (OCPs).
- *Has effect on the fetus:* Major congenital malformation (MCM) 6.4%
- *Decrease in serum concentration in pregnancy:* Up to 60–70%.

Phenobarbital
- *Mechanism of action:* Potentiation of γ-amino butyric acid (GABA)
- $t\frac{1}{2}$: 53–118 hours
- Has protein-binding action of 55%
- *Dosage:* 50–200 mg/day
- Administered once a day
- It has interaction with OCPs
- *Effect on the fetus:* MCM-6.5%, small head circumference

- *Decrease in serum concentration in pregnancy:* Up to 55%.

Carbamazepine

- *Mechanism of action:* This drug acts by modulating voltage-dependent ion channels, Na^+, Ca^{2+}, and K^+
- *t½:* 12–17 hours
- Has strong protein-binding action, i.e., 76%, hence efficacy could be low in conditions where serum albumin is low
- *Dosage:* 400–1,600 mg/day
- Administered two to three times a day
- It has interaction with OCPs
- *Effect on the fetus:* MCM 5.5%, small head circumference, microcephaly, small for gestational age (SGA), and increased chances of autistic spectrum disorders
- *Decrease in serum concentration in pregnancy:* 0–12%.

Oxcarbamazepine

- *Mechanism of action:* This drug acts by modulating voltage-dependent ion channels, Na^+, Ca^{2+}, and K^+
- *t½:* 8–15 hours
- *Protein-binding action:* 60%
- *Dosage:* 600–3,000 mg/day
- Administered two to three times a day
- Has interaction with OCPs
- *Effect on the fetus:* MCM 3%
- *Decrease in serum concentration in pregnancy:* 36–62%.

Lamotrigine

- *Mechanism of action:* This drug acts by modulating voltage-dependent ion channels, including Na^+, Ca^{2+}, and K^+
- *t½:* 15–35 hours
- *Protein-binding action:* 55%
- *Dosage:* 50–150 mg/day (when used as single or add on valproate), its dose increases to 200–500 mg/day when added onto enzyme inducing AEDs
- Administered twice a day if used as single agent or once a day if added with valproate (once daily possible with monotherapy and valproate comedication)
- *Effect on the fetus:* MCM 2.9%
- *Decrease in serum concentration in pregnancy varies from 17 to 69%.*

Levetiracetam

- *Mechanism of action:* It acts by modulation of synaptic neurotransmitter release via binding to the protein SV2A in the brain
- *t½:* 6–8 hours
- *Protein-binding action:* <10%.
- *Dosage:* 1,000–3,000 mg/day
- Administered twice a day
- Nonenzyme-inducing drug
- *Effect on the fetus:* MCM 2.4%
- *Decrease in serum concentration in pregnancy:* 40–60% with maximum decrease reached in first trimester.

Valproate

- *Mechanism of action:* It has multiple ways of action including acting on GABA levels in the central nervous system (CNS), blocking voltage gated ion channels, and inhibiting histone deacetylase
- *t½:* 6–17 hours
- Has strong protein-binding action, i.e., 90%, hence efficacy could be low in conditions where serum albumin is low
- *Dosage:* 500–2,500 mg/day
- Administered two to three times a day
- *Drug interaction:* Nonenzyme inducing
- *Has effect on the fetus:* MCM 10.4%, small head circumference, small for gestational age, increased chances of learning disorders, and autistic spectrum disorders
- *Decrease in serum concentration in pregnancy:* Up to 23%.

Topiramate

- *Mechanism of action:* Multiple modes of action mainly increasing GABA activity
- *t½:* 20–30 hours
- *Protein-binding action:* 15%
- *Dosage:* 100–400 mg/day
- Administered twice a day
- Has interaction with OCPs
- *Effect on the fetus:* MCM 3.9%, microcephaly, and small for gestational age
- *Decrease in serum concentration in pregnancy:* Up to 30%.

Pregabalin

- *Mechanism of action:* Mainly acts by blocking voltage-gated calcium channel (VGCC)
- *t½:* 5–7 hours
- *Protein-binding action:* 0%
- *Dosage:* 150–600 mg/day
- Administered two to three times a day
- *Drug interaction:* Nonenzyme inducing[6]
- *Effect on the fetus:* MCM 3.3–7.7%[7]
- *Decrease in serum concentration in pregnancy:* No evidence available.

Pharmacokinetics of Antiepileptic Drugs in Pregnancy

The state of pregnancy produces pharmacokinetic changes in women. Volume of blood increases, renal excretion increases, and liver metabolism is enhanced. By this the AEDs have an increased clearance. AED clearance is calculated by the formula:

Clearance = AED dose (mg/kg/day)/AED concentration.

Some of the AED serum concentration have been studied extensively in pregnancy. Lamotrigine, levetiracetam, and oxcarbamazepine are known to have increased clearance in pregnancy by the first trimester and hence may require an increase in the dose.

Phenobarbital, phenytoin, topiramate, and zonisamide also have reduced serum concentrations in pregnancy.

Such AEDs would require monitoring of serum levels of the AED and an increased doseduring pregnancy.

CONTRACEPTION IN WOMEN WITH EPILEPSY

Women with epilepsy need to know that the AED that they are on may interact with the OCP. The following enzyme-inducing drugs, i.e., carbamazepine, phenytoin, phenobarbital, primidone and topiramate, oxcarbamazepine, and eslicarbazepine interact with hormone-containing contraceptives those which contain estrogen, emergency contraceptive ulipristal, and even progestogen-only contraceptives. They could benefit by higher doses of estrogen like 50 µg in each tablet or changing the AED altogether as high-dose estrogen-containing contraceptives have their own adverse effects. Other contraceptive methods like copper laden intrauterine device or condoms could be used.

Alternatively nonenzyme-inducing drugs such as sodium valproate, levetiracetam, gabapentin, vigabatrin, tiagabine, and pregabalin may be prescribed. Both the Food and Drug Administration (FDA) and the European Medicine Agency (EMA) do not advise valproate in child-bearing potential women unless adequate contraceptive methods are being used.

PRECONCEPTION COUNSELING IN WOMEN WITH EPILEPSY

Women with epilepsy are anxious to know if their medications would affect the fetus. It would be prudent for the treating doctor to treat an epileptic women in reproductive age with an AED which would be least harmful for the fetus and mother. Discontinuation of AED is not advisable in pregnancy.[8]

Antiepileptic drugs have been historically said to be a cause for fetal malformations. Most commonly occurring ones are cardiac, renal, skeletal, and cleft palate. They are also said to be responsible for fetal growth restriction. AEDs have been studied for the long-term effects of the baby such as behavioral development and intelligence quotient (IQ). Valproate is known to affect both.

Carbamazepine and phenytoin have shown some decreased long-term development but not as the extent of valproate. Lamotrigine and levetiracetam have not shown long-term neurological and behavioral deficits although larger studies are required.

Changing the AED to a safer one would be considered at this stage. If epilepsy is in remission, then withdrawal of the drug could be considered. Folic acid supplementation should be considered at this stage to reduce the occurrence of neural tube defects.

Antiepileptic drugs should be given in the least effective dose. Monotherapy has been preferred. However, when polytherapy was studied in detail it was found that the specific AED used in polytherapy would be responsible for the increased malformations. Hence, it would be thought that the dose and type of the AED would be responsible for MCM. If polytherapy is to be used then the least required dose of each AED should be considered.[8]

MANAGEMENT OF WOMEN WITH EPILEPSY IN PREGNANCY

Women in pregnancy would be required to monitor the AEDs serum level at the first visit and monthly thereon. Efforts should be taken to maintain the therapeutic serum levels of the AED. In areas where the monthly levels of AED cannot be done, increasing the dose of the drug must be considered, especially in women with generalized tonic-clonic seizures and in the first trimester. Also excessive vomiting in the first trimester might lead to nonabsorption of the drug and hence a good control of vomiting should be advised. WWE are having an increased risk of sudden unexpected death in epilepsy (SUDEP) which is defined as "sudden, unexpected, witnessed or unwitnessed, nontraumatic and no drowning death in patients with epilepsy, with or without evidence for a seizure and excluding documented status epilepticus, in which postmortem examination does not reveal a toxicologic or anatomic cause for death".

Uncontrolled tonic-clonic seizures are the strongest risk factor for SUDEP, which has been seen to be the main cause of death in pregnant WWE.

Folic acid supplementation of 4 mg daily should be given in WWE as they have an increased risk of developing neural tube defects. The earlier studies have shown this increased risk as older AEDs were being used. This has not been seen with use of newer AEDs.

Screening of the WWE with nuchal translucency (NT) scan and double marker in the first trimester and targeted imaging for fetal anomaly (TIFA) in the second trimester should be advised. Fetal echo is also advisable. Serial growth reassessment scans should be done after 28 weeks of gestation.

Women with epilepsy are known to have an increased odds for abortion, antepartum hemorrhage, preterm labor, growth restriction, induction of labor, and cesarean delivery.[8]

Enzyme-inducing AEDS are said to inhibit the precursors of clotting factors that is vitamin K. Hence, vitamin K tablets were prescribed to the WWE in antenatal period. However, data suggests that this administration of vitamin K did not show to be beneficial hence it is not advised presently. The baby should receive 1 mg vitamin K intramuscularly after the delivery.

Similarly doubling the dose of antenatal corticosteroid in WWE is not advisable and regular doses of antenatal corticosteroid should be given when required.

There is 1–2% chance of having a seizure during labor and postpartum.

In the event of seizures lorazepam (4 mg bolus) is the first choice followed by diazepam (5–10 mg slow intravenous), phenytoin (10–15 mg/kg), and fosphenytoin.

Continuous cardiotocography (CTG) monitoring is preferred, especially if the woman had a seizure. There is no indication for cesarean delivery unless it is an obstetric indication. There are no contraindications for induction of labor due to interaction with AED.

During the postpartum period breastfeeding should be offered to all WWE. It does not affect the cognitive function of the baby. Sleep deprivation may lead to seizures. AED which has been increased can be reduced in the postpartum period. Care to be taken to provide adequate sleep to the WWE during the postpartum period.[9]

REFERENCES

1. Fiest KM, Sauro KM, Wiebe S, Patten SB, Kwon C-S, Dykeman J, et al. Prevalence and incidence of epilepsy: a systematic review and meta-analysis of international studies Neurology. 2017;88(3):296-303.
2. WHO. Epilepsy. [online] Available from who.int/news-room/fact-sheets/detail/epilepsy.
3. Manford M. Recent advances in epilepsy. J Neurol. 2017;264(8):1811-24.
4. Fisher RS, Cross JH, French JA, Higurashi N, Hirsch E, Jansen FE, et al. Operational classification of seizure types by the International League Against Epilepsy: Position Paper of the ILAE Commission for Classification and Terminology. Epilepsia. 2017;58(4):522-30.
5. Mula M. Third generation antiepileptic drug monotherapies in adults with epilepsy. Expert Rev Neurother. 2016;16(9):1087-92.
6. Kim H, Kim DW, Lee ST, Byun JI, Seo JG, No YJ, et al. Antiepileptic Drug Selection According to Seizure Type in Adult Patients with Epilepsy. J Clin Neurol. 2020;16(4):547-55.
7. Andrade C. Safety of Pregabalin in Pregnancy. J Clin Psychiatry. 2018;79(5):18f12568.
8. Tomson T, Battino D, Bromley R, Kochen S, Meador K, Pennell P, et al. Management of epilepsy in pregnancy: a report from the International League Against Epilepsy Task Force on Women and Pregnancy. Epileptic Disord. 2019;21(6):497-517.
9. Royal College of Obstetricians and Gynaecologists. (2016). Epilepsy in Pregnancy (Green-top Guideline No. 68). [online] Available from https://www.rcog.org.uk/guidance/browse-all-guidance/green-top-guidelines/epilepsy-in-pregnancy-green-top-guideline-no-68/.

Chapter 11

Rh Alloimmunization

Mariyam Faruqi, Devyani Misra

INTRODUCTION

Though hydrops fetalis was a recognized clinical entity as early as the 17th century, it was only in 1939 that Levine et al. discovered atypical antibodies in a case of hydrops. This was soon followed by the discovery of blood groups and the Rhesus (Rh) factor by Landsteiner and Weiner in 1940. Later, Levine et al. discovered the Rh antibody in women with pregnancies affected by hemolytic disease of the newborn (HDN). A few years later, the CDE classification was described, further widening the horizon for study of HDN.[1]

Red cell alloimmunization is the most common cause of fetal anemia. The Rh-negative mother elicits an immune response when Rh-positive fetal erythrocytes enter the circulation in significant quantity. This response in the form of Rh antibodies destroys fetal erythrocytes by transplacental passage in subsequent Rh-positive pregnancies.

Although there is risk of alloimmunization in all pregnancies of Rh-negative woman, the condition is still uncommon. Attributable reasons are insufficient amount of fetomaternal hemorrhage (FMH) to mount an immune response in the mother, low immunogenic capacity of the mother, and a coexisting maternal fetal ABO incompatibility which leads to rapid clearance of fetal erythrocytes preventing a significant maternal response.

EPIDEMIOLOGY

The documented prevalence of red cell alloimmunization in pregnancy is around 1%. In the Rh-negative population with ABO incompatibility, nearly 2% women are sensitized by the time of delivery. Another approximately 7% women are sensitized by 6 months postpartum. Nearly 7% Rh-negative will be "sensibilized" to produce antibodies in subsequent pregnancies.[2]

Without anti-D immune globulin prophylaxis, alloimmunization develops in nearly 16% of Rh-negative women with ABO-compatibility between mother and fetus. With concurrent ABO incompatibility, this figure is as low as 0.1% with prophylaxis.

GENETICS

- Rh blood group system comprises many antigens of which 5, namely, C, c, D, E, and e are immunogenic. "d" indicates absence of the D antigen. The most immunogenic D antigen defines the Rh-positive status of a person.
- The gene for Rh factor is located on short arm of chromosome 1.
- Rh-positive individuals may have either one (heterozygous) or two copies (homozygous) of the *RHD* gene whereas

Rh-negative are homozygous for complete deletion of the *RHD* gene.
- Each copy of gene is inherited from either parent, thereby implying that all offspring of a homozygous father will be Rh-positive and that of heterozygous father have a 50% chance when the mother is Rh-negative.[3]

PATHOPHYSIOLOGY

- *Maternal alloimmunization:* Throughout pregnancy, small amounts of FMHs occur repeatedly, causing circulating fetal red cells to enter maternal circulation. Rarely, the amount of bleed may be significant enough to stimulate an immune response resulting in generation of immunoglobulin M (IgM) antibody which does not cross placenta, thus sparing the ongoing pregnancy. After about 6 months of initial stimulation immunoglobulin G (IgG) antibody is produced which gets actively transported across the placenta in subsequent Rh-positive pregnancies. These bind to the fetal red cell antigens causing their sequestration and hemolysis. Rh-negative fetus is spared as it lacks the corresponding antigen.[4]

Sensitization due to passage of fetal red cells via placental route can occur antenatally in all three trimesters (7%, 16%, and 29%). Nearly 10% cases occur during pregnancy and 90% during delivery **(Box 1)**.

FETAL EFFECTS OF RH ISOIMMUNIZATION

Congenital Hemolytic Anemia

The least severe form of Rh isoimmunization, also called congenital anemia of the newborn, results from mild hemolysis of fetal red cells occurring in the baby. Mild-to-moderate anemia evolves gradually in the baby with the hemoglobin usually between 9 and 10 g/dL.

BOX 1: Causes of fetomaternal hemorrhage associated with red cell antigen alloimmunization.

Pregnancy loss
- Ectopic pregnancy
- Spontaneous abortion
- Elective abortion
- Partial molar pregnancy
- Fetal death (any trimester)

Procedures
- Chorionic villus sampling
- Amniocentesis
- Fetal blood sampling
- External cephalic version

Others
- Delivery
- Trauma
- Antepartum hemorrhage, more commonly in placental abruption
- Manual removal of placenta
- Unexplained vaginal bleeding during pregnancy
- Idiopathic

For each of the above, anti-D immune globulin is recommended

Source: The American Academy of Pediatrics and American College of Obstetricians and Gynecologists, 2012.

Jaundice is usually absent. Mild-to-moderate hepatosplenomegaly due to extramedullary hematopoiesis may develop. The condition usually settles down by 6 weeks of life due to waning of antibodies.

Icterus Gravis Neonatorum

This is a more severe form of Rh isoimmunization in which baby is usually born in good condition but jaundice appears within 24 hours of birth. During in utero stage, excess of bilirubin from fetal red cell hemolysis accumulates in body. After birth, the immature hepatobiliary system does not effectively excrete this bilirubin, leading to development of jaundice. In severe cases, kernicterus develops due to excess levels of unconjugated bilirubin crossing the blood–brain barrier with irreparable damage to the central nervous system, especially the basal ganglia and eighth cranial nerve nucleus resulting in sensorineural deafness. It usually occurs with bilirubin levels exceeding 20 mg/dL more in premature, dehydrated, and sick neonates. Anemia may be significant owing to hemolysis. Treatment includes phototherapy, adequate hydration, and exchange transfusion.[5]

Immune Hydrops or Erythroblastosis Fetalis

This is the most severe form of Rh isoimmunization. Manifestations encompass the following:
- Fetal anemia—leading to cardiomegaly and subsequent heart failure
- Neonatal hyperbilirubinemia (icterus gravis neonatorum)—serum bilirubin >20 mg/dL can lead to kernicterus
- Massive edema (hydrops fetalis) and intrauterine death.

Sequence of In Utero Events

- Maternal IgG enters fetal circulation via placenta.
- Sequestration and destruction of antibody-coated red cells occurs in the fetal liver and spleen causing *fetal anemia* (hematocrit <30%).
- Heme from hemolysed cells converted to bilirubin—*fetal hyperbilirubinemia* cleared by placenta.
- Placental enlargement with edema and large prominent cotyledons can be appreciated.
- Extramedullary erythropoiesis is stimulated with resultant *hepatosplenomegaly*. With further cell destruction, severe anemia occurs.
- Heart failure eventually ensues—*erythroblastosis fetalis with a 20–30% death rate, if untreated.*

- *Hydrops fetalis,* occurs when hematocrit falls to <15% with very high perinatal mortality rate.
- Male-to-female hydropic ratio = 3.1:1 and males are three times more likely to die.
- Ultrasound findings may show ascites, scalp and skin edema, pericardial or pleural effusion, and hepatosplenomegaly in the fetus. There may be sinusoidal pattern on cardiotocography in severe affection due to fetal anemia. Maternal X-ray abdomen though not practiced in modern era shows fetus in "Buddha position" with a halo around its head due to scalp edema.

MATERNAL EFFECTS OF RH ISOIMMUNIZATION

- Higher incidence of preeclampsia, hydramnios and fetal macrosomia. There is risk of coagulopathy and hypofibrinogenemia due to the dead retained fetus.
- Increased incidence of postpartum hemorrhage due to placentomegaly and coagulopathy.
- *Amnestic response:* Presence of an antibody titer in the mother need not necessarily depict the fetal affection. Previously sensitized women may have a higher load during subsequent pregnancies even if the fetus is D-negative.
- *The grandmother effect:* In most of pregnancies, small amount of maternal blood enters the fetal circulation. This may cause Rh-negative female fetus to become sensitized in response to maternal Rh-positive red cells. A sensitized individual may produce anti-D antibodies even before or early on in her first pregnancy and as a result HDN may develop in the first pregnancy itself. This mechanism is called the *grandmother theory* since the

fetus is jeopardized by maternal antibodies that were initially provoked by her *grandmother's* erythrocytes.[6]

ALLOIMMUNIZATION DUE TO MINOR ANTIGENS

- The routine use of anti-D immunoglobulin has brought down the cases of HDN due to D antigen and majority of cases are now reported due to other red cell antigens.
- Anti-RhD, anti-Rhc, and anti-Kell (K1) are primary cause of fetal hemolysis severe enough to require treatment with intrauterine transfusion (IUT).
- The other antigens capable of severe alloimmunization include C, E, e (Rh system: non-D); K, k (Kell system); Fya (Duffy), M (MNS), and Jka.
- Sensitization to minor antigens majorly results from incompatible blood transfusions. Red cell antibodies in pregnancy are managed similar to RhD. Alloimmunization to Kell antigen having a different pathogenesis needs different management.
  - The Lewis system antibodies, Lea and Leb, are cold agglutinins (predominantly IgM) and are not expressed on fetal red cells [The American College of Obstetricians and Gynecologists (ACOG) 2016] and thus pose no risk.[7]

Kell Alloimmunization

- Kell sensitization develops is severe and more rapidly developing compared with sensitization to D or other blood group antigens.
- Anti-Kell antibodies attach to erythrocyte precursors in the fetal bone marrow preventing normal erythropoiesis and hampering the normal response to hemolysis.
- As the erythrocytes production is impaired, the number of hemolysed red cells is less and so, severity of anemia cannot not be estimated by the maternal Kell antibody titer.
- ACOG (2016) recommends antibody titers not be used to monitor Kell-sensitized pregnancies.
- The initial management of the K1-sensitized pregnancy should involve paternal red cell typing and genotype testing.

ABO Blood Group Incompatibility

- It is the most common cause of HDN (20%) though hemolysis in the fetus is usually not severe (5%).
- ABO incompatibility usually affects firstborn neonates. Anti-A and anti-B isoagglutinins are found in most women with O blood group owing to similar antigens in bacteria causing immunization even prior to index pregnancy.
- The severity of ABO alloimmunization does not increase in successive pregnancies.
- ABO incompatibility is rarely alarming as most anti-A and anti-B antibodies are IgM and do not cross the placenta.
- Due to the relatively mild nature of the condition, intensive fetal monitoring and early delivery are not indicated in pregnancies with previous affection.
- However, neonatal observation is imperative as phototherapy may be required for hyperbilirubinemia and rarely, exchange transfusion.

MANAGEMENT OF THE ALLOIMMUNIZED PREGNANCY

Clinical Approach

Aspects of history to be explored include:
- *Rh blood type of patient and spouse:* If the father and mother are Rh-negative,

the baby will be Rh-negative and the possibility of alloimmunization does not exist.
- Prior blood transfusions
- All previous pregnancies, outcomes, and interventions. A positive history of hydrops is associated with 90% chance of recurrence.
- Previous administration of anti D prophylaxis
- Presence of vagina bleeding
- Prior invasive procedure
- *Exclusion of potentially sensitizing events:* Abortion, antipartum hemorrhage (APH), intrauterine fetal death (IUFD), multiple gestation, and manual removal of the placenta.[8]

DIAGNOSIS

- ABO blood grouping, Rh typing, and antibody screen at first prenatal visit. The presence of D antibodies in maternal serum is pathognomonic of Rh alloimmunization.
- *Indirect Coombs test (ICT):* Maternal serum is incubated with red cells and then incubated with antihuman globulin. The cells are then observed for agglutination. This is a widely used technique for determining antibodies in maternal plasma.
- When the father genotype of the father is not known, assessment of fetal genotype should be offered.
- Amniocentesis with polymerase chain reaction (PCR) testing of uncultured amniocytes has a positive predictive value (PPV) of 100% and negative predictive value (NPV) of 97%.
- Chorionic villus sampling is not preferred as it imposes a greater risk for FMH and subsequent worsening of alloimmunization.
- The novel technique of cell-free deoxyribonucleic acid (cff DNA) for fetal D genotyping from maternal plasma is now preferred as it is noninvasive fetal D with a sensitivity that exceeds 99% and with a specificity of 95%.

Kleihauer–Betke Test

This is a test for quantification of FMH.
- It is based on the principle of resistance of fetal hemoglobin (HbF) in fetal erythrocytes to acid elution compared with adult hemoglobin (HbA) in maternal cells.
- After preparation of smear and exposure to acid, HbA is denatured. On staining, the fetal cells with resistant HbF appear rose pink and the maternal cells appear as "ghosts".
- The volume of FMH is calculated as: (Maternal blood volume × Maternal hematocrit × % fetal cells in Kleihauer-Betke)

Newborn Hematocrit

In conditions of hemoglobinopathies like beta-thalassemia with elevated HbF or at term, the test is not accurate and FMH is calculated as a percentage of maternal cells.

Fetal cells in 25 high-power fields are counted and volume of FMH is calculated using following formula:

$$\frac{\text{No. of fetal cells/HPF}}{\text{No. of maternal cells/HPF}} \times 2{,}400.$$

Fetomaternal Hemorrhage

- In 2–3 per 1,000 pregnancies, the volume of FMH exceeds 30 mL of whole blood (ACOG, 2017).
- All D-negative women should be screened during pregnancy and at term using ICT. Quantitative testing performed if indicated.

- Once FMH is recognized, the volume of fetal cells transfused is calculated to estimate appropriate dose of anti D-immune globulin that should be administered. 0.1 mL fetal red blood cell (RBC) loss: 3% risk of immunization and >5 mL fetal RBC loss: 65% risk of immunization.

PREVENTION OF RHD ALLOIMMUNIZATION

- All D-negative unsensitized women are administered anti-D immunoglobulin at 28 weeks gestation and following delivery if the newborn is RhD-positive and direct Coombs test (DCT) negative.
- The half-life of anti-D immunoglobulin is 16–24 days.
- Before the 28-week dose, antibody screening is recommended to identify alloimmunization.
- Anti-D immune globulin is also recommended after pregnancy related events resulting in FMH.
- If not administered immediately following delivery, this should be given as soon as possible, as some protection occurs up to 28 days postpartum.

Mechanism of Action of Anti-D

Exact mechanism is not known. Proposed theories include clearance of anti-D coated RBCs and downregulation of specific B cells before mounting of immune response mediated by macrophages.

Dose

- RhD-negative mother and FMH with gestational age <12 weeks, 50 μg (sufficient to counter the response to 2.5 mL of Rh-positive RBC)
- For gestation >12 weeks, intramuscular dose of 300 μg or 1,500 IU provides protection against fetal hemorrhage of up to 30 mL of fetal whole blood or 15 mL of fetal red cells in an average built woman.
- Anti-D immunoglobulin administration may produce a weakly positive ICT (up to 1:4) in the mother. This is not significant and should not be regarded as alloimmunization.
- With increasing body mass index (BMI) standard doses may be less protective and increased doses may be needed.

Preparations

- Formulations are prepared by cold ethanol fractionation and ultrafiltration from human plasma of individuals with high titer anti-D immunoglobulin D antibodies.
- Anti-D should be given to all Rh-negative women who undergo termination of pregnancy (medical or surgical), ectopic pregnancy, have had tubal ligation, stillbirth delivery, or following recurrent or continued uterine bleeding for example in placenta previa.
- With immunoprophylaxis the overall risk of alloimmunization is reduced to <0.2%.
- *Anti-D at 28 weeks* reduces third trimester alloimmunization rate from 2 to 0.1%.
- Postpartum administration within 72 hours of delivery lowers risk by 90%
- Anti-D immunoglobulin should be given whenever there is doubt regarding FMH.

PREDICTION OF SEVERITY OF FETAL ANEMIA

- *First affected pregnancy:* Maternal anti-Rh antibody titers correlate well and are most useful in assessing the risk of fetal anemia.
- *Subsequent pregnancies:* The most powerful predictor is the titer at which the fetus was affected in a previous pregnancy.

Women with previous affection are at risk of developing severe fetal anemia at an earlier gestation in a subsequent pregnancy.

Timing of Intervention

- Whenever antibody level >8 IU/mL or titer more than the critical value
- 10 weeks before affection in previous pregnancy
- Earliest is at 18 weeks of gestation (fetal reticuloendothelial system is too immature to result in destruction of Ab coated RBCs prior to this).

Ultrasound Assessment

- Establish an accurate estimation of the gestational age.
- Early diagnosis of fetal hydrops characterized by an accumulation of fluid in at least two areas of the body of the fetus, polyhydramnios, or placentomegaly.
- Determine fetal growth and well-being as they are invaluable in guiding use of invasive procedures such as amniocentesis, fetal blood sampling (FBS) and IUTs.

Middle Cerebral Artery-Peak Systolic Velocity

- Middle cerebral artery-peak systolic velocity (MCA-PSV) has a sensitivity of 100% with a false positive rate of 12% for prediction of fetal anemia.
- The anemic fetus has a propensity to shunt blood preferentially to vital organs like the brain to maintain adequate oxygenation with a resultant rise in MCA-PSV owing to increased cardiac output along with decreased blood viscosity.
- Use as a screening tool permits 80% lesser requirement for invasive testing (i.e., amniocentesis and cordocentesis)
- Not useful before 18 weeks of gestation as fetal affection is infrequent.
- Less reliable indicator of severe anemia after 35 weeks due to the physiological increase in cardiac output.
- Serial measurement of the MCA-PSV is the preferred test for detection of fetal anemia.

Results

- *Unaffected/mildly affected fetus:*
  - Normal MCA-PSV: Doppler is repeated monthly. Deliver at or near term after lung maturity. Low risk of IUFD.
- *Moderately affected:*
  - MCA-PSV value 1.0–1.5 multiples of median (MoM): Surveillance includes weekly Dopplers.
- *Severely affected:*
  - MCA-PSV exceeds 1.5 MoM: If fetal gestation is <34–35 weeks, FBS and IUT should be considered as needed (Society for MFM, 2015a). MCA-PSV >1.5 MoM indicate moderate-to-severe fetal anemia with sensitivity 88% and NPV 89%. Fetus needs help to attain lung maturity before delivery as there is high risk of IUFD.

Amniotic Fluid Spectral Analysis

Liley (1961) demonstrated the utility of amniotic fluid spectral analysis to measure bilirubin concentration and to thereby estimate hemolysis severity. Amniotic fluid bilirubin concentration was measured by a spectrophotometer and was represented as the change in optical density (OD) absorbance at 450 nm—OD450. The likelihood of fetal anemia was determined by plotting the OD450 value on a graph that was divided into zones. However, the amniotic fluid bilirubin level is normally high in mid-pregnancy, limiting the reliability of this technique.

More so, this technique involved invasive procedures and with the availability of Doppler, noninvasive methods of monitoring are now preferred.

■ INTRAUTERINE TRANSFUSION

Indications

- *Severe fetal anemia:* Elevated MCA-PSV or fetal hydrops.
- Transfusion is recommended when the fetal hematocrit is <30%
- With the development of hydrops, hematocrit is usually <15%.
- Also useful in conditions of red cell alloimmunization, parvovirus B19 infections, placental chorioangioma and twin-to-twin transfusion syndrome.

Prerequisites

- Other fetal malformation complications ruled out
- Counseling of couple
- Consent
- Request for compatible blood.

Technique

- Ultrasonography (USG) guided
- No anesthesia to mother
- Spinal needle 20/22G
- *Pretransfusion sample:* Hemoglobin, hematocrit, mean corpuscular volume (MCV), blood group, and direct Coombs test
- Fresh O negative, cytomegalovirus (CMV) negative blood crossmatched against the mother and leukocyte depleted, irradiated and double packed to a hematocrit of 70–80% is used.

■ INTRAVASCULAR TRANSFUSION

The umbilical vein at the placental insertion site of umbilical cord is the commonly used site though the preferred site is the intrahepatic portion of the umbilical vein as it provides a pure fetal venous sample, avoids injury to the umbilical arteries and is associated with a reduced rate of fetal bradycardia. A 20G spinal needle is inserted under ultrasound guidance and adequate blood withdrawn for hemoglobin, hematocrit, blood grouping and typing, DCT, and reticulocyte count.

■ INTRAPERITONEAL TRANSFUSION

- Severe or early-onset hemolytic disease.
- When vascular access is not possible (fetus is <18 weeks or umbilical vein is too thin, fetus position with anterior spine, abnormal cord insertion, e.g., velamentous insertion.
- Previous failed attempt at intravascular transfusion (IVT) with cord hematoma/thrombosis.

Calculation of Volume to be Transfused

- In a nonhydropic fetus, the target hematocrit is 40–50%.
- Volume of transfusion = 0.15 × Expected fetal weight × (Expected hematocrit – Observed hematocrit)/Bag hematocrit
- Post-transfusion hematocrit is done.
- The aim of the first IUT is to raise hematocrit a only marginally above the physiological range of 35–40% before 24 weeks, 45–50% after 24 weeks, and 50–55% after 28 weeks.
- Hematocrit values decline at the rate of 1% per day after the first IUT which slows down after a second IUT usually performed after 1–2 weeks. Subsequent IUTs are performed at 3–4 weekly intervals depending on post IUT hematocrit values with an aim of maintain a hematocrit 40–45% and suppression of fetal erythropoiesis.

- In the severely anemic fetus, following the first IUT, post-transfusion hematocrit should not exceed 25% or four times the pretransfusion value. Next IUT is done after 48 hours, then after 7–10 days. Thereafter, repeat transfusions are based on hematocrit and Kleihauer–Betke stain.
- MCA-PSV can be used to monitor and predict anemia after transfusions. However, accuracy of MCA-PSV for the prediction of fetal anemia after the second IVT is not well established.

Care at Delivery

- Timing of the delivery depends on gestational age, severity of fetal anemia, and fetal maturity. If fetal surveillance is reassuring, induction of labor is done between 37 and 38 weeks.
- Steroids administered for fetal lung maturity.
- Direct agglutinin test (DAT) is performed on a cord blood in alloimmune women.
- Treatment of anemia and hyperbilirubinemia include:
  - Exchange or top-up transfusions
  - Phototherapy
  - Recombinant erythropoietin (shown to reduce the need for top-up infusions)
  - Intravenous gamma globulin.

HYDROPS FETALIS

- Condition with two or more fetal effusions—pleural, pericardial, ascites, or one effusion with anasarca.
- *Clinically significant edema:* Skin thickness >5 mm and placentomegaly (placenta thickness ≥4 cm in the second trimester or ≥6 cm in third trimester).
- Develops with a fetal hemoglobin deficit of at least 7 g/dL below the mean for the gestational age.
- It is divided into two categories, i.e., immune and nonimmune.

MANAGEMENT OF THE NEWBORN

Clinical spectrum of neonatal outcomes includes:
- Normal baby who develops mild jaundice and responds to conservative treatment.
- Normal baby who develops rapid jaundice and requires exchange transfusions.
- Baby with hydrops fetalis, anemia with hepatosplenomegaly, generalized edema, ascites, and pleural effusion. The severely affected infant may suffer perinatal asphyxia, acidosis, hypothermia, and may develop disseminated intravascular coagulation with leukopenia and thrombocytopenia. Hypoglycemia in the first 24 hours is due to hyperplasia of islet cells.
- In extreme cases there may be a stillborn baby or early neonatal death due to difficulty in establishing ventilation and perfusion.[8]

GENERAL CARE

- Cord blood should be sent for hematocrit, blood grouping and typing, DCT, bilirubin level, and reticulocyte count.
- Blood grouping may not be accurate following a recent IUT.
- In severely affected babies, serum bilirubin should be done every 6–12 hours depending on rise of bilirubin.
- Tests done for suspected kernicterus are serum albumin; serum bilirubin to albumin ratio; carboxyhemoglobin levels; bilirubin saturation index; and bilirubin reserve binding capacity.
- Early indications for exchange transfusion in such babies are cord Hb <10 g%, cord bilirubin >5 mg%, unconjugated bilirubin of 10 g% within 24 hours or 15 mg% within 48 hours.

MIRROR SYNDROME

- An association between fetal hydrops and development of maternal edema in which the fetus mirrors the mother
- *"Triple edema":* Fetus, mother, and placenta all become edematous.
- Associated with hydrops from D alloimmunization, twin-to-twin transfusion syndrome, placental chorioangioma, fetal cystic hygroma, Ebstein anomaly, sacrococcygeal teratoma, chylothorax, bladder outlet obstruction, supraventricular tachycardia, and various congenital infections.
- In most cases with mirror syndrome, prompt delivery is indicated which is soon followed by resolution of maternal edema and other findings.

REFERENCES

1. Arias F. Rh alloimmunization. In: Arias F (Ed). Practical Guide to High-risk Pregnancy and Delivery, 3rd edition. New Delhi: Harcourt India Private Ltd; 2009. pp. 358-71.
2. Royal College of Obstetricians and Gynaecologists. Anti-D Immunoglobulins for Rh Prophylaxis (Green-top Guidelines No. 22). London: Royal College of Obstetricians and Gynaecologists; 2002.
3. Royal College of Obstetricians and Gyanecologists. The Management of Women with Red Cell Antibodies during Pregnancy (Green-top Guidelines No. 65). London: Royal College of Obstetricians and Gynaecologists; 2014.
4. Leveno KJ, Spong CY, Dashe JS, Casey BM, Hoffman BL, Cunningham FG, et al. Williams Obstetrics, 25th edition. New York, USA: McGraw Hill Education; 2018. pp. 618-27.
5. American College of Obstetricians and Gynecologists. Practice Bulletin No. 181: Prevention of RhD Alloimmunization. Obstet Gynecol. 2017;130(2):e57-e70.
6. American College of Obstetricians and Gynecologists. ACOG Practice Bulletin No. 75: Management of alloimmunization during pregnancy. Obstet Gynecol. 2006; 108(2):457-64.
7. Sharma JB. Textbook of Obstetrics, 3rd edition. New Delhi: Arya Publishing Company; 2022.
8. Dutta DC, Konar H. DC Dutta's Textbook of Obstetrics, 9th edition. New Delhi: Jaypee Brothers Medical Publishers (P) Ltd.; 2021.

Chapter 12

Systemic Lupus Erythematosus in Pregnancy

Sonal Gupta

■ INTRODUCTION

Systemic lupus erythematosus (SLE) is a multisystem autoimmune disorder that most commonly affects women in their reproductive years. This is a chronic systemic connective tissue disease that flares and remissions can characterize. It can be mild or life-threatening.[1,2]

■ INCIDENCE

- According to epidemiological data, SLE prevalence in India is about 3.2 per 100,000 people.[3]
- Women are more affected than men (9:1), especially during childbearing (ratio 15:1).[1]
- It is estimated that 1 in 1,000 women are affected. The highest incidence is in Afro-Caribbean women.[1] Incidence in India is 9.9/100,000.[1]

■ CLINICAL FEATURES

- This pattern is often seen as a waxing or waning one.
- SLE can be heterogeneous and may include a range of clinical and antibody patterns.
- Joint involvement is the most common clinical feature (90%). Arthritis is a noninvasive, peripheral condition that manifests as tenderness and swelling.[4]
- Other symptoms include photosensitivity, dermal involvement, and vasculitic lesions on the fingertips and nail folds.
- Serositis may occur (pleuritis or carditis), kidney involvement (glomerulonephritis and proteinuria and cell casts) as well as neurological involvement, such as psychosis, seizures, or chorea.
- Hemolytic anemias and thrombocytopenia are some of the hematological manifestations.

■ PATHOGENESIS

- Although the cause of SLE remains unknown, it is thought to involve both genetic predispositions and environmental triggers such as ultraviolet light, demethylating medications, and infectious or exogenous viruses.
- Epstein–Barr virus was identified as a potential factor in the development of lupus.[5]
- It is possible to have polyclonal B cell activation, impaired regulation of the immune cells response by T cells, and failure to remove immune complexes.
- Nonorgan-specific antibodies are also circulating. Vasculitis is caused by the deposition of immune complexes.

■ PRECONCEPTION EVALUATION

- SLE women are more likely to become pregnant than women who are healthy.[6]
- Preconception assessments for women with SLE are essential in determining if pregnancy could pose an unusually high risk to the mother or fetus.

- It should also include a review of significant organ involvement and disease activity, as well as hypercoagulability and concurrent medical conditions that could impact pregnancy.
- It is important to inform women that stopping medications that control disease activity can increase the chance of developing lupus flares and other complications during pregnancy.
- Women planning to become pregnant should consider switching to compatible medications. This should continue throughout the pregnancy.
- It is important to review past obstetric outcomes, paying particular attention history of small fetuses, preeclampsia, and stillbirth, as well as preterm births.
- The best outcomes can be expected if SLE is inactive for at least 6 months before conception.
- Patients with active SLE, particularly nephritis should be advised not to get pregnant until the disease has been well controlled for at most 6 months.
- Pregnancy testing should include a test for antibodies to Ro/La. These antibodies could predispose you to neonatal lupus.[7]
- In extreme cases, surrogacy and adoption options should be considered.

DIAGNOSIS

- A complete blood count could show normochromic normocytic thrombocytopenia, neutropenia, and normochromic normocytic erythrocytosis.
- High levels of immunoglobulin can raise the erythrocyte sedimentation rate (ESR). Normal C-reactive protein (CRP) levels and low levels or falling off the third and fourth components of complement are indicators of active disease.
- Antinuclear antibody (ANA) is the most prevalent autoantibody in 96% of SLE patients. The titers do not change with disease activity.
- Antibodies to double-stranded deoxyribonucleic acid (DNA) are the most specific (found in 78% of patients) and Smith (Sm). These antibodies are more common in women who have glomerulonephritis.
- Patients may also have antibodies to other extractable nuclear antigens (ENAs), such as anti-Ro or anti-La, or to phospholipids.
- It is important to note that the anti-Ro and/or anti-La (present in approximately 30%) and the antiphospholipid antibodies, [antiphospholipid syndrome (APLS)—present in around 40%], are considered later.

EFFECT OF PREGNANCY ON SLE

- Pregnancy is associated with an increased risk of flare-ups of lupus.
- Studies show that flares are more common in women who are pregnant by between 25 and 65%. A recent study by Hopkins University using the Hopkins lupus cohort found that pregnant women have a 60% higher rate of flares than nonpregnant females.[8]
- Lupus flares in pregnancy usually involve the musculoskeletal or integumentary systems.[9]
- Flares can be difficult to diagnose in pregnancy because many of the features such as hair loss, fatigue, anemia, elevated ESR, and fatigue overlap with normal pregnancy.
- Prophylactic steroids cannot prevent flares. Prophylactic steroids are not recommended ante- or postpartum.
- Women with lupus may not experience a decrease in renal function during

pregnancy. However, SLE nephropathy can be present in pregnant women with lupus.

The following factors are associated with an increased risk of flare during pregnancy:[6,7,10-15]
- Flare risk is increased by the following factors
- Any active disease 6 months before conception
- A history of lupus nephritis
- Stopping hydroxychloroquine or other medications
- Primigravida pregnancy.

■ EFFECT OF SLE ON PREGNANCY

Systemic lupus erythematosus affects pregnant women who are pregnant. Pregnant women with SLE experience a two- to fourfold increase in obstetric complications, including preeclampsia and preterm birth, spontaneous miscarriage, preeclampsia, premature delivery, fetal deaths, intrauterine growth restrictions (IUGRs), thrombosis, and thrombocytopenia.[16,17]

Preeclampsia

Preeclampsia is a common complication of pregnancy in SLE and occurs in between 16 and 30% of cases. SLE affects 2% of women.[18] Preeclampsia risk factors include lupus or lupus, specific disease markers, antiphospholipid antibodies, and thrombocytopenia.

Preeclampsia presents a unique challenge because of the close resemblance between lupus and preeclampsia. Both are characterized by deteriorating renal function and increased proteinuria, hypertension, and decreased platelet counts. Preeclampsia may have elevated serum uric acid which can help distinguish the two.

Preterm Birth

Preterm birth is the most common complication of lupus. It occurs in about one-third of patients. Preterm birth is possible due to increased clinical and serological disease activity, high prednisolone usage, hypertension, and thyroid diseases. A study by Clowse et al.[19] also found elevated serum uric acids to be linked with preterm births.

The outcome of pregnancy is especially affected by kidney disease. Even quiescent renal disease is associated with a higher risk of fetal loss, preeclampsia, and IUGR, especially if there is hypertension or proteinuria.

Preeclampsia and pregnancy loss are similar to the general population in women in remission but without hypertension, renal involvement, or APLS.

Chorea is a rare complication of pregnancy for women with SLE/APLS.

Neonatal Lupus

This is a temporary condition that can last from 6 to 8 months after birth. It is caused by passively acquired autoimmunity due to maternal antibodies that cross over the placenta. They last until the maternal antibodies are gone from fetus circulation. It usually manifests as a raised red rash and other hematologic or hepatic abnormalities. It can also be associated with structural abnormalities, cardiac conduction defects, cardiomyopathy, and congestive heart disease in its worst form.[20-22]

It is seen in approximately 10% of patients with positive SSA (anti–Ro) or SSB (anti–La) antibodies.

Complete Heart Block

This is the most serious complication of neonatal lupus. This happens in approximately 2% of newborns whose mothers have SSA/SSB antibodies.

If a previous infant has been affected by neonatal lupus, the risk is higher. It can reach 16–18% for one child and 50% for two. The effect on subsequent infants is similar to their siblings.

MANAGEMENT DURING PREGNANCY

A multidisciplinary team of rheumatologists, obstetricians, and specialists in high-risk pregnancy care can best provide care for patients with SLE.

This should begin with periconceptional counseling. The chances of a successful pregnancy are better if it occurs in the midst of remission from the disease.

Monitor SLE activity: Women should have their disease activity checked by a rheumatologist at least once per trimester. If they have an active condition, it is recommended that they be evaluated more often.

Initial Evaluation

Examine including:
- Blood pressure
- Complete blood count (CBC)
- Renal function (urea, electrolytes, and creatinine)
- Urinalysis spot urine protein/creatinine
- Tests of liver function
- Anti-Ro/SSA, anti-La/SSB antibody testing if they have not been evaluated previously
- Antiphospholipid antibodies [lupus anticoagulant (LA), anticardiolipin (aCL) antibody, and anti-β_2 glycoprotein antibodies]
- Anti-β_2-glycoprotein (GP)
- Anti-double-stranded DNA antibodies (dsDNAs)
- Complement (CH 50 or C3 and/or C4).

It is then recommended to take serial measurements at different intervals, depending on the severity of the disease.

Maternal and Fetal Monitoring

- It is unknown what the optimal monitoring schedule should be to ensure fetal and maternal well-being during pregnancy. Fetal monitoring is an option for women with SLE **(Table 1)**.
- To determine the expected date of delivery, a first trimester ultrasound evaluation is performed. At 18 weeks of gestation, a detailed fetal anatomic survey is done.
- Ultrasound evaluation of fetus growth and a placental deficiency during the third trimester. The frequency of monitoring fetus growth will vary depending on

TABLE 1: Antenatal monitoring in SLE pregnancy.

Clinical review	Investigations	Specific monitoring
• Rheumatologist: Four to six times weekly, more frequently if there is an active disease or flare • Monthly until week 20, then weekly until week 28, then weekly thereafter	• Every visit: Blood count and serum uric acid, creatinine, urea, creatinine; electrolyte levels; liver function tests; urinalysis; spot urine protein/creatinine ratio; complement levels • Ultrasound: Early pregnancy to check for fetal anomalies. 4 weeks thereafter to monitor fetal growth. Weekly form week 26	• Fetus echocardiography: Positive anti-Ro antibodies, weekly starting at week 16–26, and biweekly thereafter, continuing until delivery • Preeclampsia: Uterine arterial Doppler study (week 20, 4 weekly thereafter), fetal umbilical artery Doppler velocity (weekly starting week 26) • IUGR: Increased frequency of ultrasound and FST growth monitoring

(FST: fetal surveillance tests; IUGR: intrauterine growth restriction; SLE: systemic lupus erythematosus)

maternal and fetal health, but it is usually performed every 4 weeks.
- Fetal surveillance using nonstress tests (NSTs) and/or biophysical profiles during the last 4–6 weeks is recommended for women with lupus.
- Patients with positive anti-R0/SSA or anti-La/SSB antibody levels should be monitored more closely for any cardiac problems.
- Preeclampsia symptoms in these patients should be monitored closely.

Postpartum Surveillance

Postpartum disease may be exacerbated in some women. Women with active disease or significant end-organ damage at the time of conception are more likely to experience flare-ups during their postpartum period than women who had no disease.

DIFFERENTIATION OF LUPUS NEPHRITIS FROM PREECLAMPSIA

This can be extremely difficult and may result in two conditions being combined. Preeclampsia can mimic lupus flares in pregnancy. This includes increased proteinuria, hypertension, and thrombocytopenia. Sometimes, evidence of lupus activity can be seen in other organs. This can help to distinguish between SLE and preeclampsia.

Preeclampsia can be distinguished from lupus or flare by laboratory testing. However, this is not always the case.
- Preeclampsia has no proteinuria, but lupus nephritis can be associated with proteinuria (proteinuria) and/or active urine sediment (red cells, white cells, and cellular casts).
- Flares of SLE may be related to low or declining complement levels and higher titers of anti-DNA antibodies. In contrast, preeclampsia[23,24] has normalized or increased complement levels.[23]
- Preeclampsia is more likely to be caused by hyperuricemia or abnormal liver function tests.
- Renal biopsy is the only way to distinguish a renal flare from preeclampsia. However, this is very rare in pregnancy.
- Preeclampsia and lupus flare cannot be distinguished beyond 24–28 weeks of gestation. If the fetus viability is not assured, then delivery may be an option. Preeclampsia can be treated by delivery. It will also allow for the administration of drugs like cyclophosphamide to treat a renal flare.

■ TREATMENT

To care for a pregnant woman with SLE, a rheumatologist, a skilled obstetrician with high-risk care, and a nephrologist should be part of a team.

Periconceptional Counseling

This should be done in conjunction with periconceptional counseling. Knowing the anti-Ro/La status, APLS and renal function can help to predict the risks for the woman and her fetus.

If conception is performed during the remission of the disease, the outcome will be better. It is important to review and adjust medications with the goal of maintaining good disease control and ensuring safety for the mother and fetus.

It is important to assess thyroid function as hypothyroidism in SLE can lead to poorer outcomes.

Prepregnancy counseling should include a discussion about appropriate medication use during pregnancy. Unfortunately,

TABLE 2: Medications safe for use during systemic lupus erythematosus (SLE) pregnancy.

Drugs	Comments	Recommendations
Nonsteroidal anti-inflammatory drugs (NSAIDs)	First-trimester use may be associated with a higher risk of congenital malformations, fetal renal impairment, and premature closure of ductus arteriosus with use in last trimester	• Use with caution during the first and second trimester • Discontinue during last trimester
Corticosteroids • Prednisolone/pulse methyl-prednisolone fluorinated compounds (betamethasone/dexamethasone)	• High doses can lead to higher maternal complications • Some association with impaired neuropsychological development of the child	• Use lowest possible dose • Pulse therapy can be used for acute flares • Limit to one course, for fetal lung maturation
Antimalarials • Hydroxychloroquine	Reduced risk of disease flares, congenital heart block (CHB), and neonatal lupus syndrome (NLS)	Should be continued in all SLE pregnancies
Immunosuppressants • Azathioprine • Calcineurin inhibitors (cyclosporine/tacrolimus)	Used in a large number of transplant recipients. The recent report of late developmental delays in offsprings with azathioprine	• Limit azathioprine dose to 2 mg/kg/day • Explain the probability of late effects in the child to mother
Antihypertensives • Methyldopa • Labetalol Nifedipine • Hydralazine	Concerns about growth retardation with labetalol and impaired uteroplacental blood flow with hydralazine	Generally safe and preferred drugs for hypertension during pregnancy

discontinuation of therapy due to concerns about presumed toxicity can lead to an increase in disease activity and worsening outcomes. Although most SLE therapies are contraindicated and potentially dangerous, there are safe options that can be used during pregnancy **(Table 2)**.

During the first and second trimesters, nonsteroidal anti-inflammatory drugs (NSAIDs) were considered safe.[25] Recent research has shown that there are moderate associations between NSAIDs and certain birth defects in the first trimester.[26,27] The use of NSAIDs after 20 weeks gestation is associated with an increased risk for impaired fetus renal function. NSAIDs should be used cautiously during pregnancy. Continued use of NSAIDs after the 32nd week can increase the likelihood of premature closing of the ductus arteriosus almost 15-fold.

This should be avoided.[28] There is limited data available on the effects of cyclooxygenase-2 inhibitions during pregnancy. They should be avoided.

Limiting your exposure to steroids during pregnancy is a good idea. Doses that are too high during pregnancy can increase the risk of preeclampsia and diabetes.[25] In the event of severe disease flares, you can use short courses of high doses or intravenous pulses of methylprednisolone.

Long-term steroid therapy patients should be administered stress doses at delivery. In cases of premature delivery, the use of fluorinated compounds such as betamethasone or dexamethasone should be restricted to one course for fetus lung maturation.[29]

All pregnant women suffering from SLE should continue taking hydroxychloroquine. Numerous studies have shown the positive effects of hydroxychloroquine during pregnancy in SLE. Use during pregnancy was associated with a reduction in disease activity and no adverse effects on the baby while discontinuing use led to an increase in disease flares.[30] In pregnancies at high risk for congenital heart block (CHB) or neonatal lupus, the risk of developing CHB and other complications was significantly lower when continued use of hydroxychloroquine was maintained.[31]

Azathioprine, one of the few immunosuppressive drugs that have been proven safe during pregnancy, is the most widely used. To avoid fetus cytopenia or immune suppression, the maximum daily dose should not exceed 2 mg/kg/day. The calcineurin inhibitors (tacrolimus and cyclosporine) and cyclosporine have not been linked to an increase in fetal mortality. Other agents such as methotrexate and cyclophosphamide should be stopped at least 3 months before conception.

Pregnancy is a time when most commonly prescribed antihypertensive medications must be avoided (or used with extreme caution).[32-34] Angiotensin-converting enzyme (ACE) inhibitors and angiotensin II receptor blockers can cause specific malformations, such as the ACE-inhibitor fetopathy. Additionally, neonatal arterial hypotension and renal failure have been reported. IUGR and fetal bradycardia have been linked to β-adrenergic blocking medications. Diuretics can cause maternal volume loss and decreased uteroplacental flow. The safe arsenal against hypertension in pregnancy is very limited. It includes drugs such as nifedipine, hydralazine, and methyldopa.[33,34]

Aspirin is a low-dose antiplatelet agent and is safe for pregnant women, but there is not much data.[34] Heparin is safe and does not cross the placenta. It is therefore the preferred anticoagulant during pregnancy. Low-molecular-weight heparin, also known as LMWH, has the same safety and efficacy as unfractionated heparin (UFH). LMWH is more popular than UFH because of its ease of administration, better antithrombotic/anticoagulant ratio, and predictable bioavailability.[35]

All pregnant women with SLE should receive calcium supplementation, particularly those who are taking corticosteroids or heparin. Low levels of vitamin D during pregnancy can lead to higher rates of pregnancy morbidity, including preeclampsia and gestational diabetes. Supplemental vitamin D in pregnancy did not significantly or consistently lower the risk.[36]

Breastfeeding is safe for lupus patients after pregnancy. Prednisolone, hydroxychloroquine, and azathioprine have very little transfer to breast milk so they can be continued while you are breastfeeding.

■ CONCLUSION

Lupus patients have had their pregnancy outcomes improve over the years. However, there is still a higher risk of having a baby with lupus and a greater chance of developing lupus flares. To ensure a successful outcome for both mother and baby, it is important to have a thorough understanding of the pathophysiologic process and to be able to monitor and manage pregnancy from multiple perspectives.

■ REFERENCES

1. Rees F, Doherty M, Grainge M, Davenport G, Lanyon P, Zhang W. The incidence and prevalence of SLE in the UK, 1999–2012. Ann Rheum Dis. 2016;75(1):136-41.
2. Dall'Era M. Systemic Lupus Erythematosus. In: Dall'Era M (Ed): Current Diagnosis and Treatment: Rheumatology, 3rd edition. New York, United States: McGraw Hill; 2013.

3. Malaviya AN, Singh RR, Singh YN, Kapoor SK, Kumar A. Prevalence of Systemic Lupus Erythematosus in India. Lupus. 1993;2:115-8.
4. Branch DW, Khamashta MA. Antiphospholipid syndrome: obstetric diagnosis, management, and controversies. Obstet Gynecol. 2003;101(6):1333-44.
5. Stagnaro-Green A, Akhter E, Yim C, Davies TF, Magder L, Petri M. Thyroid disease in pregnant women with systemic lupus erythematosus: increased preterm delivery. Lupus. 2011;20:690-9.
6. Buyon JP, Kim MY, Guerra MM, Laskin CA, Petri M, Lockshin MD, et al. Predictors of Pregnancy Outcomes in Patients with Lupus: a Cohort Study. Ann Intern Med. 2015;163: 153-63.
7. Ruiz-Irastorza G, Khamashta MA. Lupus and pregnancy: ten questions and some answers. Lupus. 2008;17:416-20.
8. Eudy AM, Siega-Riz AM, Engel SM, Franceschini N, Howard AG, Clowse MEB, et al. Effect of pregnancy on disease flares in patients with systemic lupus erythematosus. Ann Rheum Dis. 2018;77:6:855-60.
9. Petri M. The Hopkins Lupus Pregnancy Center: ten key issues in management. Rheum Dis Clin North Am. 2007;33:227-35.
10. Clowse ME, Magder LS, Witter F, Petri M. The impact of increased lupus activity on obstetric outcomes. Arthritis Rheum. 2005;52:514-21.
11. Yang H, Liu H, Xu D, Zhao L, Wang Q, Leng X, et al. Pregnancy related systemic lupus erythematosus: clinical features, outcome and risk factors of disease flares—a case-control study. PLoS One. 2014;9:e104375.
12. Kwok LW, Tam LS, Zhu T, Leung YY, Li E. Predictors of maternal and fetal outcomes in pregnancies of patients with systemic lupus erythematosus. Lupus. 2011;20:829-36.
13. Clowse ME, Magder L, Witter F, Petri M. Hydroxychloroquine in lupus pregnancy. Arthritis Rheum. 2006;54(11):3640-7.
14. Gladman DD, Tandon A, Ibañez D, Urowitz MB. The effect of lupus nephritis on pregnancy outcome and fetal and maternal complications. J Rheumatol. 2010;37(4):754-8.
15. Saavedra MA, Sánchez A, Morales S, Navarro-Zarza JE, Ángeles U, Jara LJ. Primigravida is associated with flare in women with systemic lupus erythematosus. Lupus. 2015;24(2):180-5.
16. Smyth A, Oliveira GH, Lahr BD, Bailey KR, Norby SM, Garovic VD. A systematic review and meta-analysis of pregnancy outcomes in patients with systemic lupus erythematosus and lupus nephritis. Clin J Am Soc Nephrol. 2010;5(11):260-8.
17. Petri M. Prospective study of systemic lupus erythematosus pregnancies. Lupus. 2004;13(9):688-9.
18. Chakravarty EF, Colón I, Langen ES, Nix DA, El-Sayed YY, Genovese MC, et al. Factors that predict prematurity and preeclampsia in pregnancies that are complicated by systemic lupus erythematosus. Am J Obstet Gynecol. 2005;192(6):1897-904.
19. Clowse ME, Wallace DJ, Weisman M, James A, Criscione-Schreiber LG, Pisetsky DS. Predictors of preterm birth in patients with mild systemic lupus erythematosus. Ann Rheum Dis. 2013;72(9):1536-9.
20. Vanoni F, Lava SAG, Fossali EF, Cavalli R, Simonetti GD, Bianchetti MG, et al. Neonatal Systemic Lupus Erythematosus Syndrome: a Comprehensive Review. Clin Rev Allergy Immunol. 2017;53(3):469-76.
21. Klein-Gitelman MS. Neonatal Lupus: What We Have Learned and Current Approaches to Care. Curr Rheumatol Rep. 2016;18(9):60.
22. Brito-Zerón P, Izmirly PM, Ramos-Casals M, Buyon JP, Khamashta MA. The clinical spectrum of autoimmune congenital heart block. Nat Rev Rheumatol. 2015;11(5): 301-12.
23. Buyon JP, Cronstein BN, Morris M, Tanner M, Weissmann G. Serum complement values (C3 and C4) to differentiate between systemic lupus activity and pre-eclampsia. Am J Med. 1986;81(2):194-200.
24. Clowse ME, Magder LS, Petri M. The clinical utility of measuring complement and anti-dsDNA antibodies during pregnancy in patients with systemic lupus erythematosus. J Rheumatol. 2011;38(6):1012-6.

25. Lateef A, Petri M. Managing lupus patients during pregnancy. Best Pract Res Clin Rheumatol. 2013;27(3):435-47.
26. Hernandez RK, Werler MM, Romitti P, Sun L, Anderka M. Nonsteroidal anti-inflammatory drug use among women and the risk of birth defects. Am J Obstet Gynecol. 2012;206(3):228.e1-8.
27. Adams K, Bombardier C, van der Heijde DM. Safety of pain therapy during pregnancy and lactation in patients with inflammatory arthritis: a systematic literature review. J Rheumatol Suppl. 2012;90:59-61.
28. Koren G, Florescu A, Costei AM, Boskovic R, Moretti ME. Nonsteroidal anti-inflammatory drugs during the third trimester and the risk of premature closure of the ductus arteriosus: a meta-analysis. Ann Pharmacother. 2006;40(5):824-9.
29. Wapner RJ, Sorokin Y, Mele L, Johnson F, Dudley DJ, Spong CY, et al. Long-term outcomes after repeat doses of antenatal corticosteroids. N Engl J Med. 2007;357(12):1190-8.
30. Levy RA, Vilela VS, Cataldo MJ, Ramos RC, Duarte JL, Tura BR, et al. Hydroxychloroquine (HCQ) in lupus pregnancy: double-blind and placebo-controlled study. Lupus. 2001;10(6):401-4.
31. Izmirly PM, Costedoat-Chalumeau N, Pisoni CN, Khamashta MA, Kim MY, Saxena A, et al. Maternal use of hydroxychloroquine is associated with a reduced risk of recurrent anti-SSA/Ro-antibody-associated cardiac manifestations of neonatal lupus. Circulations. 2012;126(1):76-82.
32. Ostensen M, Lockshin M, Doria A, Valesini G, Meroni P, Gordon C, et al. Update on safety during pregnancy of biological agents and some immunosuppressive anti-rheumatic drugs. Rheumatology. 2008;47 Suppl 3:iii28-31.
33. American College of Obstetricians and Gynecologists. ACOG Practice Bulletin No. 125: Chronic hypertension in pregnancy. Obstet Gynecol. 2012;119(2 Pt 1):396-407.
34. Mustafa R, Ahmed S, Gupta A, Venuto RC. A comprehensive review of hypertension in pregnancy. J Pregnancy. 2012;2012:105918.
35. Giannubilo SR, Tranquilli AL. Anticoagulant therapy during pregnancy for maternal and fetal acquired and inherited thrombophilia. Curr Med Chem. 2012;19(27):4562-71.
36. De-Regil LM, Palacios C, Ansary A, Kulier R, Pena-Rosas JP. Vitamin D supplementation for women during pregnancy. Cochrane Database Syst Rev. 2012;2:CD008873.

Chapter 13
Hepatitis B Infection in Pregnancy

Padma Shukla, Sonal Agrawal

■ INTRODUCTION

Viral infection may be present during pregnancy or it may occur before pregnancy and women may conceive during the disease course. Hepatitis B infection is one of them and it leads to a significant burden on healthcare system. Two billion people are affected with the hepatitis B virus (HBV)[1] in all over world. 350–400 million people are clinically infected with the HBV.[2] Acute hepatitis B infection occur in 2 per 1,000 pregnant women. Majority of new diagnosis are due to mother-to-child transmission.[3] HBV infection causes short-term and long-term sequelae in the neonates and in mother. Acute hepatitis B infection incidence is same in pregnant and in nonpregnant women.

■ ETIOLOGY

Hepatitis B virus belongs to the Hepadnaviridae family. It is small, enveloped, and hepatotropic virus. HBV is a double-standard deoxyribonucleic acid (DNA) virus having four proteins; surface protein [hepatitis B surface antigen (HBsAg)], core protein [hepatitis B core antigen (HBcAg)], DNA polymerase, and X protein.

Hepatitis B virus can be detected in serum 1–2 months after exposure. Incubation period is of 45–160 days. HBsAg appears before clinical evidence of the disease. HBsAg level remains elevated during symptomatic phase of acute hepatitis and beyond. Hepatitis B surface antibody (HBsAg) develops in resolving phase of infection and provides long-term immunity. HBcAg is confined to the liver cells and it is not detectable routinely in the serum.

Acute and chronic HBV infection can be diagnosed by detection of the anti-HBc immunoglobulin M (IgM), which predominates during first 6 months after acute infection. Immunoglobulin G (IgG) anti-HBc antibody is present beyond 6 months of infection. Hepatitis B e antigen (HBeAg) is the other marker which appears simultaneously or shortly after appearance of HBsAg. HBeAg indicates the high level of virus replication and the presence of high viral load. Presence of antibody to e antigen correlates with the lower infectivity.[4]

■ EPIDEMIOLOGY

Modes of hepatitis B transmission are sexual contact, parenteral, mucosal exposure to blood and vertical transmission from mother to child.[5] Newborns are mostly infected if the mother contract the infection during the third trimester or is a chronic carrier. If an acute maternal infection occurs in first trimester, the risk of vertical transmission is very less. When infection occurs in second and third trimester, risk of newborn infection is 10% and 90%, respectively.[6] Most perinatal transmission occurs in intrapartum period (95%). Vertical transmission depends on the antigen and antibody status of the mother, if mother is HBsAg positive and HBeAg positive risk of vertical transmission is 70–90%. If mother is positive for HBsAg risk of infection is 25% but presence of HBsAg and hepatitis B e antibody (HBeAb) in mother lead to less chance of (10–15%) vertical transmission.[7]

Risk of development of chronic HBV infection is 2–6% in adults. HBV carrier is the most important factor in HBV transmission. A patient who is HBV positive on two occasions at 6 months apart is known as carrier.

■ EFFECT ON PREGNANCY

Hepatitis B virus is not teratogenic. Acute viral hepatitis B is associated with increased risk of spontaneous miscarriage and preterm labor. It also causes low birth weight in neonates. There could be possibility of intrapartum and postpartum hemorrhage if the prothrombin time is prolonged. Chronic HBV infection progression is not affected by pregnancy.

■ DIAGNOSIS

Hepatitis B infection can be diagnosed by serological tests for the hepatitis B virus antigen (HBsAg and HBeAg) and antibodies to HBsAg, HBcAg, and HBeAg. Clinical presentation and determination of the serological pattern can evaluate stages of hepatitis B infection.

The sign and symptoms of acute hepatitis B is flu-like illness. Symptoms appear gradually, fatigue, anorexia, nausea, and vomiting are predominating symptoms. Myalgia, malaise, headache, and pharyngitis may be other clinical features. Jaundice with low grade fever may be present. Jaundice can persist for 4–6 weeks. Signs of hepatomegaly, splenomegaly, and lymphadenopathy may appear in 10–20% of the cases. The severity of the disease is directly correlated with signs and symptoms. Slow resolution of symptoms occurs. Complete recovery is seen in majority of the patients. The chronic carrier stage will develop in some of the patients. Chronic disease symptom may vary from inactive state to recurrent exacerbation chronic hepatitis; cirrhosis, and hepatocellular carcinoma.[8]

There are more chances of development of chronic hepatitis in infants (90% cases) exposed to HBV infection. Children clear the virus in 50% cases.[9] 5% adult progress to chronic disease. Recent studies revealed that CXCL13, a B lymphocyte is expressed in an age dependent manner in human hepatic macrophages. This lymphocyte is responsible for an immune response to control the virus.[10]

Chronic hepatitis B progresses through four phases. Immune tolerance is the first phase, viral clearance is seen in second phase, inactive carrier state is the third phase, and hepatitis B is reactivated in the fourth phase. It is difficult to characterize patient disease status.

■ LABORATORY TEST

A universal screening of all pregnant women for hepatitis B (HBsAg) during each pregnancy must be done. Characteristics of all phases is mentioned in **Table 1**. HBV DNA testing for HBsAg-positive pregnant women along with HBeAg is required. Various antigenic tests suggest different phase of viral infection.

- HBsAg—marker of infection (current)
- IgM anti-HBc—recent infection (first 6 months)
- IgG anti-HBc—past infection
- HBe antigen—it is a marker of active replication and infectivity
- HBV DNA—it is a marker of viral load and guide the need of antiviral therapy
- Anti-HBs—marker of resolved infection prevention of perinatal transmission.

TABLE 1: Characteristics of the phases of HBV infection.[6]

Phase	HBeAg	HBV DNA	ALT	Liver histology	Indication for treatment
Immune-tolerant	Positive	Elevated: >200,000 IU/mL	Normal	Minimal inflammation and fibrosis	No
• HBeAg-positive • Immune-active	Positive	≥20,000 IU/mL	Elevated >2 × ULN	Moderate-to-severe inflammation or fibrosis	Yes
Inactive CHB	Negative	Low or undetectable	Normal	Minimal inflammation, variable fibrosis	No
HBeAg-negative reactivation phase	Negative	Elevated: ≥ 2,000 IU/mL	Elevated	Moderate-to-severe inflammation or fibrosis	Yes

(ALT: alanine aminotransferase; CHB: chronic hepatitis B; HBeAg: hepatitis B e antigen; HBV: hepatitis B virus; DNA: deoxyribonucleic acid; ULN: upper limit of normal)

PREVENTION OF PERINATAL TRANSMISSION

Vertical transmission of hepatitis B infection can be prevented by following measures:
- Screening of all antenatal women routinely.
- Women at risk for contracting HBV infection counsel them about vaccination.
- Liver infection and viral load is advised for women who test positive for HBsAg.[11]
- Evaluation of household contacts is recommended and those are not infected should be vaccinated.
- All healthcare providers should be vaccinated and should take standard precaution against exposure to blood.
- All newborn babies should receive hepatitis B vaccine and immunoglobulin (HBIG) and within 12 hours of birth. This therapy is 85–95% effective in prevention of the HBV chronic carrier state in neonates.
- The Centers for Disease Control and Prevention (CDC) advises vaccination of all infants born to HBsAg-negative mothers.[12]

TREATMENT

Supportive care is the key for acute HBV infection. Measurement of HBV DNA at baseline and 28 weeks along with HBeAg and alanine aminotransferase (ALT) levels is recommended. Referral to a specialist is required if viral load is >20,000 IU/mL, ALT is >19 IU/mL or HBeAg is positive.[13,14] If viral load is less or HBeAg is negative then referral can be done postpartum. Women with high viral load >200,000 IU/mL should be considered for antiviral therapy at 32 weeks to reduce viral load prior to delivery. Antiviral therapy is also given if patients are suffering from active liver disease with low viral load. Reduced viral load prevents vertical transmission.

ANTIVIRAL THERAPY

In present scenario, treatment is based on disease stage, HBV viral load, serological status, and degree of liver injury. Mothers with high viral load, HBIG, and HBV vaccination fail to prevent vertical transmission in up to 30% of children.[15] There is direct correlation between maternal predelivery HBV DNA levels and immune-prophylaxis failure.[16] Postnatal transmission of HBV is rare.

The American College of Gastroenterology (ACG) and the American Association for the Study of Liver Diseases (AASLD) guidelines advise for antiviral therapy at 28–32 weeks of pregnancy in women with high viral load. Tenofovir and telbivudine remain first-line therapy. Antiviral therapy with tenofovir in high viral load mothers improves maternal ALT levels, decreases infant HBV DNA at birth, and decreased HBV DNA positivity at 6 months.[17] Tenofovir 30 mg/day or telbivudine 600 mg/day can be given. Tenofovir is continued till 6 weeks postpartum. Lamivudine is the other drug recommended in the third trimester. It reduces resistance development and fetal exposure in the dose of 100 mg per day.

The duration of treatment is 0–3 months in postpartum period, depending on the indication for treatment initiation, HBS positivity, and breastfeeding.

Woman of childbearing age group with chronic hepatitis B, usually remain in early stage of the disease therefore antiviral therapy is not required. Patients with high viral load may be treated from antiviral therapy when they plan to become pregnant. Patient with significant liver disease including fibrosis and cirrhosis should be placed on antiviral drugs.

Peginterferon 180 g/week is the only finite treatment available for chronic hepatitis B. Women who become pregnant on antiviral therapy may require discussion of the risk of antiviral discontinuation against fetal exposure. Antiviral therapy may be continued in a pregnant female with decompensated cirrhosis.

MODE OF DELIVERY AND BREASTFEEDING

Cesarean section should not be performed for the sole indication of reducing vertical HBV transmission.[18] Cesarean should be done only for obstetric indication. Fetal scalp electrodes and fetal scalp blood sampling should be avoided. According to the World Health Organization (WHO) there is no additional sign of HBV transmission through breastfeeding even in the absence of immunization.

Postpartum Management

Active and passive immunization of the neonate should be offered at birth followed by three doses of hepatitis B vaccine. If infant has not received vaccination with in first 7 days, then three-dose course of combination vaccine should be given, at 2, 4, and 6 months of age. Anti-HBsAg antibody and HBsAg should be measured at 3–12 months after completing the vaccine course in infants born to mothers with chronic hepatitis B.[18]

Chronic hepatitis B women on antiviral therapy in pregnancy should be evaluated in postpartum period for hepatitis B flares. Hepatitis B positive women should be on lifelong follow up to prevent complications such as liver disease and hepatocellular carcinoma.

CONCLUSION

Acute hepatitis B infections during pregnancy need symptomatic and supportive care in most of the patients. Complete recovery occurs in majority of patients. The American College of Obstetricians and Gynecologists (ACOG) recommends referral to a specialist if viral load is >20,000 IU/mL, ALT >19 IU/mL, or HBeAg is positive. If patient is carrier and in immune tolerant phase, no treatment will be required. Women with immune active phase, with cirrhosis, or women who had previous child with failed passive active immunization, antiviral therapy is recommended.

REFERENCES

1. Zuckerman AJ, editor. Hepatitis B in the Asian Pasific Region. Vol. 1 3. London: Royal College of Physicians;1999.
2. Terrault NA, Bzowej NH, Chang KM, Hwang JP, Jonas MM, Murad MH, et al.

AASLD guidelines for treatment of chronic hepatitis B. Hepatology. 2016;63:261-83.
3. Tram TT. Hepatitis B in pregnancy. Clin Infect Dis. 2016;62(Suppl 4):S314-7.
4. Dinstag JL, Warts JR, Koff RS. Acute hepatitis. In: Baunwald E, Isselbacher KJ, Petersdorf RG, Wilson JD, Martin JB, Fauci AS (Eds). Harrison's Principles of Internal Medicine, 10th edition. New York: McGraw Hill; 1987. pp. 1325-35.
5. Jonas MM, Reddy RK, De Medina M, Schiff ER. Hepatitis B infection in a large Municipal obstetric population; characterization and prevention of perinatal transmission. Am J Gastroenterol. 1990;85:277-80.
6. Benjaminov FS, Heathcote J. Liver disease in pregnancy. Am J Gastroenterol. 2004;99:2479-88.
7. Beasley RP, Hwang LY, Lee GC, Lan CC, Roan CH, Huang FY, et al. Prevention of perinatally transmitted hepatitis B virus infection with hepatitis B immune globulin and hepatitis B vaccine. Lancet. 1983;2:1099-102.
8. Gish RG, Gadano AC. Chronic hepatitis B: current epidemiology in the Americas and implications for management. J Viral Hepat. 2006;13:787-98.
9. Alter MJ. Epidemiology of hepatitis B in Europe and worldwide. J Hepatol. 2003;39 Suppl 1:S64-9.
10. Publicover J, Gaggar A, Nishimura S, Van Horn CM, Goodsell A, Muench MO, et al. Age-dependent hepatic lymphoid organization directs successful immunity to hepatitis B. J Clin Invest. 2013;123(9):3728-39.
11. Petermann S, Ernest JM. Intrapartum hepatitis B screening. Am J Obstet Gynecol. 1995;173(2):369-73.
12. Centers for disease control. Hepatitis B Virus: A Comprehensive Strategy for Eliminating Transmission in the United States Through Universal Childhood Vaccination: Recommendations of the Immunization Practices Advisory Committee (ACIP). MMWR. 1991;40(RR-13):1-19.
13. American College of Obstetricians and Gynecologists. ACOG Practice Bulletin No. 86: viral hepatitis in pregnancy. Obstet Gynecol. 2007;110(4):941-56.
14. Nguyen G, Garcia RT, Nguyen N, Trinh H, Keeffe EB, Nguyen MH. Clinical course of hepatitis B virus infection during pregnancy. Aliment Pharmacol Ther. 2009;29(7):755-64.
15. Pan CQ, Duan ZP, Bhamidimarri KR, Zou HB, Liang XF, Li J, et al. An algorithm for risk assessment and intervention of mother to child transmission of hepatitis B virus. Clin Gastroenterol Hepatol. 2012;10(5):452-9.
16. Zou H, Chen Y, Duan Z, Zhang H, Pan C. Virologic factors associated with failure to passive–active immunoprophylaxis in infants born to HBsAg-positive mothers. J Viral Hepat. 2012;19(2):e18-25.
17. Chen HL, Lee CN, Chang CH, Ni YH, Shyu MK, Chen SM, et al. Efficacy of maternal tenofovir disoproxil fumarate in interrupting mother-to-infant transmission of hepatitis B virus. Hepatology. 2015;62(2):375-86.
18. Society for Maternal-Fetal Medicine (SMFM); Dionne-Odom J, Tita AT, Silverman NS. #38: Hepatitis B in pregnancy screening, treatment, and prevention of vertical transmission. Am J Obstet Gynecol. 2016;214(1):6-14.

14

Urinary Tract Infection in Pregnancy

Mamta

■ INTRODUCTION

Urinary tract infections (UTIs) are one of the most common types of infections found in pregnant women. In some women, UTI may be present before conception, e.g., the woman may have the renal stone or calculi in any part of ureter or in the bladder. Due to the physiological changes that occur in renal system may predispose the urinary tract infection, especially pyelonephritis in pregnant woman.[1]

Urinary tract infection in pregnancy can be divided into three categories:
1. Acute cystitis
2. Acute pyelonephritis
3. Asymptomatic bacteriuria (ASB).

All these three types of infection during pregnancy may lead to bad fetal and maternal outcome if left untreated. That is why it is recommended that screening of all pregnant women must be done for ASB and other infections in urinary tract. Those women who are positive for screening must be treated with proper antibiotics. In pregnancy, recurrent infection in urinary tract is also high so in this condition prophylactic antibiotic must be given.

Group B streptococcal infection may lead to serious complications during pregnancy both maternal and fetal, thus it should be treated with prophylactic antibiotics.

Acute pyelonephritis is the most serious type of all UTIs in pregnancy and it may lead to high mortality and morbidity both in mother and neonates.

It is important to understand about the normal and abnormal changes found in renal system and in urinary tract during pregnancy. Proper evaluation and adequate treatment of all cases of UTIs in pregnancy should be done for better outcome.

■ EPIDEMIOLOGY

Urinary tract infection is very common in pregnancy. About 2–7% of pregnant women may develop ASB and 1–4% of pregnant women may have the complain of acute cystitis. ASB is the main predisposing factor for developing UTI in pregnant women. If ASB is left untreated or not given adequate treatment, it may lead UTIs in around 25% of cases. Multiparous women and women belonging to low socioeconomic status are more prone for ASB. It is recommended that ASB screening must be done in first antenatal visit in all pregnant women and must be screened for ASB at the first prenatal visit. The most appropriate method to screen the ASB is to take a clean catch urine sample and send it for culture and sensitivity test. According to the culture report ASB must be treated with antibiotics.

The other factors that may lead to UTIs are:
- Young age
- Previous history of UTI
- Anemia
- Multiparity.

ETIOPATHOGENESIS

Pregnancy is an immune compromised state and there are higher chances of having infections including UTIs also.

Due to the hormonal changes (estrogen and progesterone) there are some changes that happen in kidneys, ureter, and urinary bladder during pregnancy. These changes are both anatomical as well as functional. These changes starts soon after conception and it may persist even after delivery. Women are at increased risk for UTIs. Pregnancy is associated with significant anatomic and functional changes in the kidney and its collecting system. Anatomic changes begin shortly after conception and may persist for several months after delivery. Dilatation of renal pelvis and ureter occurs in almost 90% of pregnant women due to variation in the hormones of pregnancy and pressure effect of gravid uterus. The other changes in urinary tract system are increased volume of urinary bladder and decreased tone of ureters. This may lead to stasis of urine and increased ureterovesical reflux. As plasma volume increases during pregnancy, this leads to decrease in urinary concentration. Approximately 70% of pregnant women may have the glycosuria. This causes increase in growth of bacteria in urine. Increases in urinary progestins and estrogens may lead to a decreased ability of the lower urinary tract to resist invading bacteria.

BACTERIOLOGY

The main organism which causes UTI in pregnancy is *Escherichia coli* (80–90%).

The other pathogens that may be responsible for developing UTI in pregnancy are:
- *Streptococcus faecalis*
- *Klebsiella pneumoniae*
- *Proteus mirabilis*
- *Enterococcus* species.

The pathogens or bacterial species are almost same both in pregnant and nonpregnant women.

SIGNS AND SYMPTOMS

Most of the patients of UTIs are asymptomatic. Some women may have the history of recurrent UTI or presence of ASB in her previous pregnancy.

The common symptoms of UTIs in pregnancy are:
- Painful micturition
- Burning sensation during urination
- Increase frequency of urination
- Urgency
- Supra pubic pain
- Fever >100°F or 38°C
- Chills and rigors
- Flank pain.

Some nonspecific symptoms are feeling of nausea, malaise, weakness, decrease appetite, and sometimes vomiting. In severe infection, sign and symptoms of sepsis may be present such as tachycardia and hypotension. Urinary sepsis requires proper evaluation and timely interventions.

SCREENING OF URINARY TRACT INFECTION IN PREGNANCY

All pregnant women should be screened twice during pregnancy for ASB.

According to the *American College of Obstetrics and Gynecology (ACOG)*, culture of urine must be done at the first antenatal visit and in the third trimester culture of urine must be repeated.

The *US Preventive Services Task Force* recommended that urine culture should be done between 12 and 16 weeks of gestation.

Asymptomatic Bacteriuria

Asymptomatic bacteriuria is most commonly defined as high level growth of a single bacterial organism (>100,000 colonies per milliliter) on urine culture of a specimen collected in an appropriate fashion from an individual without symptoms or signs referable to urinary infection.[2]

Asymptomatic bacteriuria means presence of rapidly multiplying bacteria within the urinary tract in pregnant women. The incidence varies from 2 to 7% depending upon the characteristic population. ASB may be present before conception so screening to be done in all pregnant women at her first antenatal visit. If the urine culture is found positive then it should be treated with proper antimicrobial drugs.[3]

Oral Antimicrobial Agents Used for Treatment of Pregnant Women with Asymptomatic Bacteriuria (Table 1)[5]

Previously, ampicillin was the drug of choice, but due to increase resistance of ampicillin for *E. coli* now it is not very effective drug for treatment of UTI in pregnancy.

Nowadays, nitrofurantoin is the highly effective drug in UTIs, especially for *E. coli*. Penicillin and cephalosporins are safe in pregnancy.

Cystitis and Urethritis

This refers to infection of urinary bladder and urethra during pregnancy. Bladder infection usually present as dysuria, increase frequency, and urgency of urination. In some cases, pyuria and bacteriuria may be found. In cases of hemorrhagic cystitis, there may be hematuria also. In around 40% of cases, it may involve the upper urinary tract also (ascending infection).

Most of the cystitis can be treated by giving 3 days antibiotic course. In some cases, coinfection of *Chlamydia trachomatis* may be present. Mucopurulent discharge from cervix may be found and can be effectively treated by azithromycin.

Acute Pyelonephritis

Acute pyelonephritis is defined as bacterial infection of the urinary tract and kidneys. It is one of the most deadly complications found in pregnant women. It complicates about 0.5–2% of all pregnancies.[4] In some cases it may lead to septic shock in pregnancy. In preterm infants, this infection causes increase incidence of cerebral palsy.

Clinical Findings

Acute pyelonephritis develops more frequently in the second trimester. The other risk factors are:
- Nulliparity
- Young age
- Pregestational diabetes.

TABLE 1: Antimicrobial agents used for treatment of pregnant women with asymptomatic bacteriuria.

Antibiotic	Dose	Duration
• Amoxicillin	• 500 mg orally QID or 875 mg orally BD	• 5–7 days
• Cefpodoxime	• 100 mg orally 12 hourly	• 5–7 days
• Cephalexin	• 500 mg orally 6 hourly	• 5–7 days
• Nitrofurantoin	• 100 mg orally 12 hourly	• 5–7 days

(*Source:* Landon M, Galan H, Jauniaux E, Driscoll D, Berghella V, Grobman W, et al. Gabbe's Obstetrics Normal and Abnormal Pregnancies, 8th edition. Amsterdam, Netherlands: Elsevier; 2020.)

Usually pyelonephritis is found unilateral and it is more common in right side of renal tract (>50%) but it can be bilateral also (25%).

The presenting symptoms are:
- Fever >100.4° or 38.5°C
- Chills with rigors
- Pain at flank area
- Vomiting.

Some common general symptoms are anorexia, nausea, vomiting, etc. On examination tenderness found at costovertebral angle. If in any case we are suspecting pyelonephritis, the urine sample should be collected by catheterization to avoid contamination from lower genital tract infection. On urine microscopic examination, there may be pus cells, white blood cells (WBCs), and bacteria. In some rare conditions (2%), some patient may present with respiratory distress syndrome due to lung injury caused by endotoxin release. These endotoxins released in blood may lead to hemolysis which causes anemia also.

MANAGEMENT

- Hospitalization should be done.
- Urine cultures should be obtained if the fever is >39°C.
- Adequate hydration should be maintained by giving intravenous fluids.
- Renal function tests (RFTs), especially serum creatinine, should be checked if we are giving any nephrotoxic drugs.
- Obtain blood cultures if the temperature is >39°C.
- Urinary output must be maintained at rate of >50 mL/hour, if not adequate intravenous crystalloid solution should be given.
- Acetaminophen is the ideal drug to be given to lower the high grade temperature. Pregnant women in her first trimester are high risk for developing teratogenic effect from hyperthermia.
- Chest X-ray is advised only in case of severe dyspnea and tachypnea.
- Complete blood count (CBC) and RFT should be repeated in next 48 hours.
- Once the patient becomes afebrile, intravenous antibiotic to be changed into oral form.
- After completing the treatment, urine culture should be repeated.

Treatment regimens for pyelonephritis are given in **Table 2**.[5]

PERSISTENT INFECTIONS

Generally, these patients respond well on intravenous antibiotics and intravenous fluid. But in some patients the infection may persist for longer duration.

If the fever does not subsided after 48–72 hours of if it reoccurs one should check for urinary tract obstruction or any another complication. To rule out any obstruction at renal system, ultrasonography (USG) of

TABLE 2: Treatment regimens for pyelonephritis.

Antibiotic	Intravenous dose	Comment
• Ceftriaxone	• 1 g 24 hourly	• Common first-line agent
• Cefepime	• 1 g 12 hourly	• Covers pseudomonas
• Aztreonam	• 1 g 8 hourly	• Useful option in women with beta lactam allergy
• Ampicillin plus gentamicin	• 1–2 g 4–6 hourly or • 1.5 mg/kg 8 hourly	• Other agents preferred to avoid aminoglycoside exposure
• Piperacillin-tazobactam	• 3.375 g 6 hourly	• Useful for severe infection

(*Source:* Landon M, Galan H, Jauniaux E, Driscoll D, Berghella V, Grobman W, et al. Gabbe's Obstetrics Normal and Abnormal Pregnancies, 8th edition. Amsterdam, Netherlands: Elsevier; 2020.)

kidneys, ureter, and bladder (KUB) area to be done. In USG of KUB, there may be any renal or ureteric calculi, abnormal dilatation in ureter, or pyelocalyceal dilatation.[6]

In some rare cases, the persistence infection can be due to abscess at perinephric area or phlegmon. To relieve the obstruction, cystoscopy-guided double-J ureteral stenting should be done. In some very serious complicated case, stone removal by surgery may be required.

CONCLUSION

Interprofessional collaboration is crucial in the management of these ill patients. With the administration of antibiotics patients may show initial worsening due to the release of endotoxin, however, most patients improve within 72 hours. Long-term complications such as renal damage are rare.

REFERENCES

1. Gilstrap LC, Ramin SM. Urinary tract infections during pregnancy. Obstet Gynecol Clin North Am. 2001;28(3):581-91.
2. Patterson TF, Andriole VT. Bacteriuria in pregnancy. Infect Dis Clin North Am. 1987;1:807-22.
3. Lucas MJ, Cunningham FG. Urinary infection in pregnancy. Clin Obstet Gynecol. 1993;36(4):855-68.
4. Wing DA, Fassett MJ, Getahun D. Acute pyelonephritis in pregnancy: an 18-year retrospective analysis. Am J Obstet Gynecol. 2014;210(3):219.e1-6.
5. Landon M, Galan H, Jauniaux E, Driscoll D, Berghella V, Grobman W, et al. Gabbe's Obstetrics Normal and Abnormal Pregnancies, 8th edition. Amsterdam, Netherlands: Elsevier; 2020.
6. Cunningham FG, Leveno KJ, Bloom SL, Dashe JS, Hoffman BL, Casey BM, et al. Williams Obstetrics, 25th edition. New York, United States: McGraw Hill; 2018.

Chapter 15

Dengue in Pregnancy

Richa Sharma, Ajay Adhikari

■ INTRODUCTION

Dengue fever is an arthropod borne viral illness which causes significant mortality and morbidity across the world including in pregnant females. It is commonly referred to as breakbone fever or seven day fever. The culprit organism is a single stranded ribonucleic acid (RNA) virus that belongs to *Flavivirus* family and has four different serotypes (DENV 1-4). Infection with any one of these serotypes provides lifelong immunity to that individual from that particular serotype.[1] *Aedes* mosquito that transmits the virus is commonly found in tropical countries such as India, which is why dengue is one of the leading causes of pyrexia in pregnant females in India. Despite rapid urbanization, an upward trend has been seen in the incidence dengue over past few decades.[2] This chapter will give insights on how this deadly disease further complicates pregnancy and how to effectively manage dengue in pregnancy.

■ EPIDEMIOLOGY

Majority of people affected by dengue are asymptomatic or have mild symptoms due to which its prevalence is highly underreported.[3] One study estimates around 390 million dengue infections across world every year out of which 96 million present with varying severity of symptoms.[4] Although there are no accurate figures depicting the burden of disease in pregnant females, it is known to cause adverse maternal and fetal outcomes. The reporting of dengue to the World Health Organization (WHO) has increased by more than eight times in couple of decades due to better communication between healthcare facilities and health ministries.

■ PATHOPHYSIOLOGY

Once the virus is injected into intradermal tissue following the bite of mosquito, skin macrophages and dendritic cells are known to be its primary targets. These cells are then believed to reach lymph nodes from where they spread to other organs via lymphatic system. Symptom onset occurs after a phase of viremia which lasts up to 48 hours. Patient's immune response to virus play a key role in determining whether the infection will be asymptomatic or progress to severe dengue with increased microvascular permeability and shock. **Figure 1** summarizes pathophysiology of dengue virus.

■ MATERNAL TRANSMISSION

Although mosquito vectors are most common mode of transmission of dengue virus, there is some evidence of transmission by pregnant mother to her baby as well. However, rate of vertical transmission is found to be low and often linked with the timing of dengue

Dengue in Pregnancy

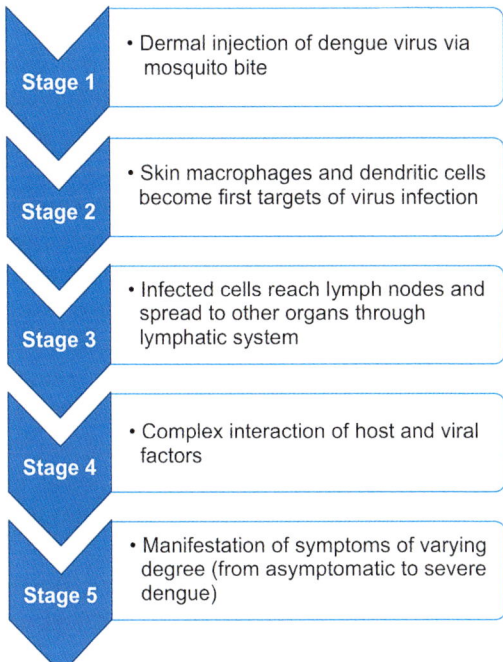

Fig. 1: Pathophysiology of dengue virus.

BOX 1: Clinical phases of dengue fever.

Febrile phase
- It is characterized by high grade fever which is sudden in onset and reaches approximately 40°C
- Fever typically lasts for 2–7 days and is continuous or saddleback in type[7]
- Associated symptoms generally include erythema, myalgia, arthralgia, headache, nausea, and vomiting

Critical phase
- It lasts up to 2 days and is characterized by defervescence. There is increased capillary permeability in this phase
- Decreased platelet count and increased hematocrit are common laboratory findings
- Special attention to warning signs must be given in this phase. Warning signs which indicate toward severe disease and increased risk of mortality include abdominal pain or tenderness, persistent vomiting, ascites, pleural effusion, mucosal bleed, and hepatomegaly

Recovery phase
- The fluid leaked in extravascular compartments due to capillary leak is slowly reabsorbed
- Bradycardia may be observed

infection during the course of pregnancy.[5] Incidence of maternal transmission is significant if infection occurs within 5 weeks of delivery. A positive correlation between pregnant female with dengue fever and complications such as preterm birth, low-birth-weight, and fetal distress has also been established.[6]

CLINICAL FEATURES

Spectrum of the disease may vary from being asymptomatic to undifferentiated fever to hemorrhagic complications to shock. Incubation period generally lasts from 2 to 7 days followed by prodromal phase of headache and malaise.

Dengue fever is generally divided into three phases as depicted in **Box 1**.

In severe dengue, organs such as liver, kidney, heart, central nervous system (CNS) and other isolated organs may be involved further complicating the disease and increasing mortality. Dengue hemorrhagic fever, disseminated intravascular coagulation, dengue shock syndrome, acute respiratory distress syndrome (ARDS), encephalitis and myocarditis are few of the life-threatening complications.

Thorough assessment of pregnant females is vital because their symptoms of dengue may be similar to preeclampsia.

WORLD HEALTH ORGANIZATION CASE DEFINITION OF DENGUE

The disease is classified in following case definitions for the purpose of better identification and prompt initiation of treatment.[8] **Box 2** depicts the WHO case definition of dengue.

> **BOX 2:** WHO case definition of dengue.
>
> *Probable dengue fever*
> - Exposure in endemic area
> - Fever
> - Any two of following—nausea/vomiting, rash, aches/pains, positive tourniquet test, leukopenia, or any warning sign
>
> *Dengue with warning signs*
> - Probable dengue with one of the following—abdominal pain or tenderness, persistent vomiting, signs of fluid accumulation, mucosal bleed, hepatomegaly >2 cm, rapid rise in hematocrit, and fall in platelet count
>
> *Severe dengue*
> - Severe plasma leakage leading to shock (dengue shock syndrome) or respiratory distress
> - Severe hemorrhagic complications
> - Sever organ involvement (liver, CNS, kidney, cardiomyopathy, pancreatitis, acute lung injury, and DIC)
>
> (CNS: central nervous system; DIC: disseminated intravascular coagulation; WHO: World Health Organization)

CHALLENGES IN DIAGNOSIS OF DENGUE DURING PREGNANCY

Hemodilution is normal physiological process during pregnancy but it hampers with diagnosis of dengue and its complications. Hemodilution masks thrombocytopenia, leukopenia, and increased hematocrit levels which are early laboratory markers of severe dengue.[9] A few common obstetric conditions are known to cause elevation of liver enzymes which further creates confusion as it is also a marker of hepatic involvement in dengue. Pregnancy being a hypercoagulable state may also lead to misdiagnosis of some other complications of dengue like disseminated intravascular coagulation or dengue hemorrhagic fever.[10] Vomiting which is a warning sign of severe dengue may also be easily misconstrued as hyperemesis during pregnancy.

LABORATORY DIAGNOSIS

Various virus isolation methods and serological methods play key role in diagnosis of the disease. Different techniques may be used at different time of presentation. During first week of infection, virus can be isolated by reverse transcriptase-polymerase chain reaction (RT-PCR). Another method is detection of NS1 antigen on rapid diagnostic test kits, which is cheaper and requires less skill. Serological methods like enzyme-linked immunosorbent assay (ELISA) detect antidengue antibodies. Immunoglobulin M (IgM) antibodies are detected from 1 week to 3 months of infection while IgM antibodies are detected from months to years.

Patient presenting during first week of illness should be tested for both virus isolation by RT-PCR or NS1 detection and serological evaluation.

Once diagnosed it should be kept in mind that dengue is a notifiable disease and must be reported to local health bodies.

DIFFERENTIAL DIAGNOSIS

Other causes of pyrexia in pregnancy must always be excluded before making the final diagnosis. Malaria, chikungunya, influenza, and measles are few other common causes of pyrexia in pregnancy. Detailed history, immunization, travel history, and history of exposure to mosquitoes are important to reach the diagnosis. Sometimes serological tests may show false positive results due to infection from other *Flavivirus* such as yellow fever and *Zika* virus.

ADVERSE MATERNAL OUTCOMES IN DENGUE WITH PREGNANCY

Various studies have established increased risk of adverse maternal and fetal outcomes in pregnant females with dengue infection. Organ dysfunction or multiorgan failure is found to be associated with poor prognosis in pregnant as well as nonpregnant females with dengue,[11] hence special attention and intensive care unit (ICU) care must be given to pregnant female suffering from dengue with any clinical or laboratory evidence suggesting organ failure such as acute kidney injury, hepatic failure, and ARDS. Elevated liver enzymes or serum creatinine are independent risk factors of poor prognosis in dengue with or without pregnancy.[12]

Previous studies have indicated that there is no significant increase in rate of cesarean section in pregnant females with dengue.[13] Although marked increased risk of postpartum hemorrhage (PPH) due to dengue-related thrombocytopenia has been observed. Rate of PPH in dengue with pregnancy is fairly high (anywhere between 2 and 30% of all deliveries).[14] Hence, intense monitoring of pregnant female with dengue in third stage of labor along with timely and judicious transfusion of blood components is important.

A positive correlation has also been found between dengue and pregnancy and risk of miscarriage in a prospective case control study conducted in 2012.[15] The rate of stillbirth in pregnant female with dengue is estimated to be between 3.8 and 13.1% as per various studies;[16] however, exact mechanism of this increased rate of stillbirth is not yet understood. Whether this increase in incidence of stillbirth is due to hyperthermia or dengue virus itself is yet to be analyzed in future studies.

ADVERSE FETAL OUTCOMES IN DENGUE WITH PREGNANCY

Just like mother dengue in pregnancy can be equally hazardous for the health of fetus. Various complications to fetus should come in mind of obstetrician managing pregnant female suffering from dengue. Dengue-related hyperthermia has been linked to increased risk of congenital malformations in fetus, such as neural tube defects.[17] Preterm birth and low-birth-weight are some other adverse outcomes for fetus that have shown positive correlation with dengue in pregnancy.[18] A meta-analysis in 2016 again reiterated increased risk of low-birth-weight and preterm births in dengue with pregnancy.[19] The reason for these adverse events is believed to be due to maternal illness rather than direct effect of the virus on the fetus. Mothers with severe dengue and complications like hemorrhagic fever showed greater risk of adverse fetal outcomes. There is also a very high chance of preterm birth within 10 days of onset of symptoms in mothers suffering from dengue.

Not all studies have shown such devastating consequences for the baby but still there is enough evidence in literature for the treating obstetricians to be alarmed by the situation. Considering all the maternal and fetal risks we have discussed earlier, it becomes imperative to manage all symptoms and complications of dengue in pregnancy timely and promptly.

MANAGEMENT OF DENGUE IN PREGNANCY

Before beginning the management part it is important to note that dengue at any stage of pregnancy is in no way an indication for termination of pregnancy. The most important part of management of dengue fever is identification of onset of critical phase. Clinically evident effusion or ascites indicates that the critical phase has already begun several hours ago. The onset of critical phase

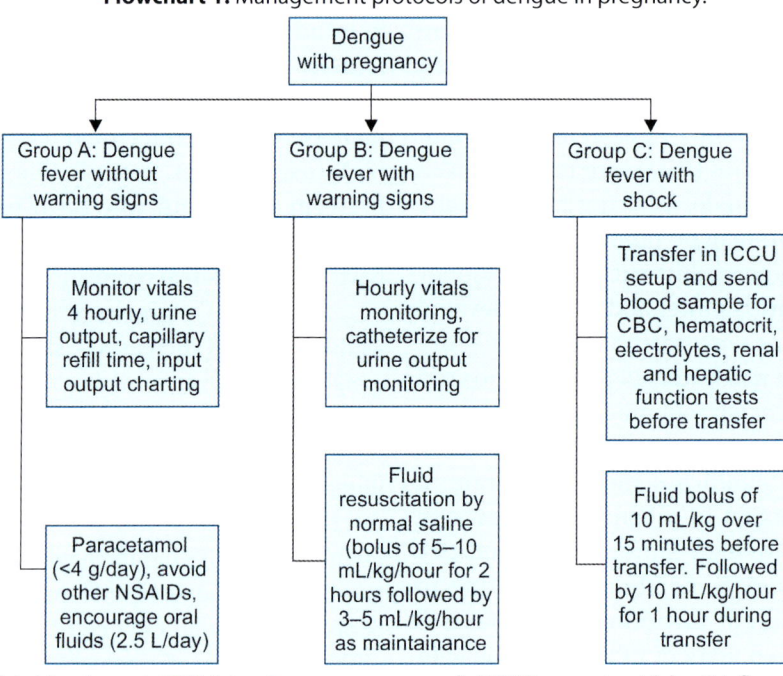

Flowchart 1: Management protocols of dengue in pregnancy.

(CBC: complete blood count; ICCU: intensive coronary care unit; NSAIDs: nonsteroidal anti-inflammatory drugs)

can be accurately depicted by beginning of rise in hematocrit levels.[20] Declining platelet counts also indicate that patient has risk of landing in critical phase in next 24 hours.

It is imperative that all pregnant females with suspected or confirmed dengue fever be admitted in hospital for close monitoring purpose. For the purpose of proper management patients are divided into three groups. Management protocols are summarized in **Flowchart 1**.

Dengue fever without warning signs should be managed by encouraging oral fluids and paracetamol. Use of other nonsteroidal anti-inflammatory drugs (NSAIDs) like ibuprofen or diclofenac must be avoided. In case of dengue fever with warning signs or dengue fever with shock, normal saline is the fluid of choice for resuscitation and is preferred over ringer lactate or dextrose sodium chloride solution (DNS). Use of colloids in dengue fever with shock is justified if there is no clinical improvement after two bolus of crystalloids.

Prophylactic platelet transfusion is not indicated; however, if delivery is inevitable within 6 hours, transfusion can be done to maintain platelet count over 50,000 per µL for normal delivery and over 75,000 per µL for cesarean section. Similarly, blood loss should be recognized and whole blood or packed cell transfusion should be initiated before blood loss exceeds 500 mL. Oxytocin infusion to prevent PPH is common practice in dengue with pregnancy to avoid excessive blood loss. Operative delivery should be performed purely for obstetric indications and planned induction surgery must be avoided. There is no role of use of steroids, immunoglobulins, or prophylactic antibiotics.

It is suitable to discharge the patient only when she is afebrile for >1 day, hematocrit levels are normal and platelet counts are in rising trend.

CONCLUSION

Dengue is one of the leading causes of pyrexia in pregnancy and has the potential to complicate the pregnancy and adversely affect maternal and fetal health. Past two decades have seen alarming increase in the incidence of dengue with or without pregnancy. The severity of disease depends very much upon the patient's immune response to virus. Majority of patients are asymptomatic or have mild symptoms at presentation. Special attention must be given to warning signs as they indicate severe disease with fatal complications. Symptoms and signs of dengue may often be confused with preeclampsia and some other physiological events during pregnancy, hence detailed history and timely laboratory investigation helps clinch the diagnosis. Due to heightened risk of adverse maternal and fetal complications such as PPH, low-birth-weight, and preterm delivery management protocols should be followed precisely in dengue with pregnancy. Use of fluids and blood components should be prompt and judicious. All pregnant patients with dengue must be managed in inpatient department (IPD) and be discharged only when they are afebrile for 24 hours, platelet counts are on rising trend, and risk of complications have subsided after critical phase.

REFERENCES

1. Seixas G, Salgueiro P, Bronzato-Badial A, Gonçalves Y, Reyes-Lugo M, Gordicho V, et al. Origin and expansion of the mosquito Aedes aegypti in Madeira Island (Portugal). Sci Rep. 2019;9(1):2241.
2. Sharma M, Glasner DR, Watkins H, Puerta-Guardo H, Kassa Y, Egan MA, et al. Magnitude and functionality of the NS1-specific antibody response elicited by a Live-attenuated tetravalent dengue vaccine candidate. J Infect Dis. 2020;221(6):867-77.
3. Waggoner JJ, Gresh L, Vargas MJ, Ballesteros G, Tellez Y, Soda KJ, et al. Viremia and clinical presentation in nicaraguan patients infected with zika virus, chikungunya virus, and dengue virus. Clin Infect Dis. 2016;63(12):1584-90.
4. Bhatt S, Gething PW, Brady OJ, Messina JP, Farlow AW, Moyes CL, et al. The global distribution and burden of dengue. Nature. 2013;496(7446):504-7.
5. Basurko C, Matheus S, Hildéral H, Everhard S, Restrepo M, Cuadro-Alvarez E, et al. Estimating the risk of vertical transmission of dengue: a prospective study. Am J Trop Med Hyg. 2018;98(6):1826-32.
6. Pouliot SH, Xiong X, Harville E, Paz-Soldan V, Tomashek KM, Breart G, et al. Maternal dengue and pregnancy outcomes a systematic review. Obstet Gynecol Surv. 2010;65(2):107-18.
7. Ng DH, Wong JG, Thein TL, Leo YS, Lye DC. The Significance of Prolonged and Saddleback Fever in Hospitalised Adult Dengue. PLoS One. 2016;11(12):e0167025.
8. Wharton-Smith A, Green J, Loh EC, Gorrie A, Omar SFS, Bacchus L, et al. Using clinical practice guidelines to manage dengue: a qualitative study in a Malaysian hospital. BMC Infect Dis. 2019;19(1):45.
9. Malhotra N, Chanana C, Kumar S. Dengue infection in pregnancy. Int J Gynecol Obstet. 2006;94:131-2.
10. Basurko C, Carles G, Youssef M, Guindi WEL. Maternal and foetal consequences of dengue fever during pregnancy. Eur J Obstet Gynecol Reprod Biol. 2009;147:29-32.
11. Padyana M, Karanth S, Vaidya S, Gopaldas JA. Clinical profile and outcome of dengue fever in multidisciplinary intensive care unit of a Tertiary level Hospital in India. Indian J Crit Care Med. 2019;23:270-3.
12. Saroch A, Arya V, Sinha N, Taneja RS, Sahai P, Mahajan RK. Clinical and laboratory factors associated with mortality in dengue. Trop Doct. 2017;47:141-5.

13. Tan PC, Rajasingam G, Devi S, Omar SZ. Dengue infection in pregnancy: prevalence, vertical transmission, and pregnancy outcome. Obstet Gynecol. 2008;111: 1111-7.
14. Tien Dat T, Kotani T, Yamamoto E, Shibata K, Moriyama Y, Tsuda H, et al. Dengue fever during pregnancy. Nagoya J Med Sci. 2018; 80:241-7.
15. Tan PC, Soe MZ, Lay KS, Sm W, Sekaran SD, Omar SZ. Dengue infection and miscarriage: a prospective case control study. PLoS Negl Trop Dis. 2012;6:e1637.
16. Carles G, Talarmin A, Peneau C, Bertsch M. Dengue fever and pregnancy. A study of 38 cases in French Guiana. J Gynecol Obstet Biol Reprod. 2000;29:758-62.
17. Edwards MJ. Review: hyperthermia and fever during pregnancy. Birth Defects Res A Clin Mol Teratol. 2006;76:507-6.
18. Xiong YQ, Mo Y, Shi TL, Zhu L, Chen Q. Dengue virus infection during pregnancy increased the risk of adverse fetal outcomes? An updated meta-analysis. J Clin Virol. 2017;94:42-9.
19. Paixão ES, Teixeira MG, Costa M, Rodrigues LC. Dengue during pregnancy and adverse fetal outcomes: a systematic review and meta-analysis. Lancet Infect Dis. 2016;16:857-65.
20. Ministry of Health. National Guidelines on Management of Dengue Fever and Hemorrhagic Fever in adults and children. Colombo, Sri Lanka: Ministry of Health; 2011.

Chapter 16

HIV in Pregnancy

Indira Palo

INTRODUCTION

The first human immunodeficiency virus (HIV) case in India was detected in 1986, when 10 samples from 102 female sex workers in Chennai tested positive. With 40.1 million (33.6–48.6 million) deaths caused by HIV to date, it is still a significant worldwide public health concern.[1] HIV infection cannot be cured, but with more people having access to good HIV prevention, diagnosis, treatment, and care, it has evolved into a chronic illness that can be managed, allowing those who have it to live long and healthy lives.

EPIDEMIOLOGY

According to the Joint United Nations Programme on HIV/AIDS (UNAIDS) 2021 global report, there are an estimated 37.6 million (30.2–45 million) persons living with HIV (PLHIV) with significant regional variation in PLHIV statistics. Globally, about 1.5 million (1.1–2.1 million) persons contracted HIV in 2020, and of them, 690,000 (480,000–1 million) people died from acquired immunodeficiency syndrome (AIDS)-related diseases. Antiretroviral treatment (ART) was provided to an estimated 27.4 million (26.5 to 27.7 million) people living with HIV worldwide in 2020.[2] Despite this remarkable accomplishment, the biggest problem right now is getting the remaining PLHIV on ART in order to lower mortality, comorbidities, and stop HIV from spreading.

According to the India HIV estimation report 2020, the national adult (15–49 years) HIV prevalence was estimated to be 0.22% (0.17–0.29%) in 2020; among men, it was 0.23% (0.18–0.31%), and among females, it was 0.20% (0.15–0.26%).[3] According to the report, between 1,533,000 and 2,908,000 pregnant women needed ART to prevent mother-to-child transmission (MTCT) of HIV. A major commitment made under the National AIDS Control programme (NACP) is to prevent MTCT of HIV. Though considerable, the development on eliminating mother-to-child transmission (EMTCT) is still far from the goal, according to HIV estimate 2020. Between 2010 and 2020, there was a 55% decrease in new HIV infections among children annually, which is a significant accomplishment. According to estimates, the overall MTCT rate (including the breastfeeding period) in 2020 will be about 27.4% (20.3–33.5%), down from over 40.2% in 2010. However, compared to the desired target of 5%, the MTCT rate continues to be higher than average.[3]

ETIOPATHOGENESIS OF AIDS

Human immunodeficiency virus is the virus that causes AIDS. HIV has two primary strains: HIV-1 and HIV-2. Both can lead to AIDS. HIV-2 occurs in a much smaller number of people, mostly in West Africa. In the US, it makes up only 0.01% of all HIV cases, and those are primarily people from

West Africa.[4] The HIV attacks the immune system and diminishes people's resistance to a variety of illnesses and cancers that healthy immune systems are better able to resist. Infected individuals eventually lose their immunological capacity as the virus kills and damages immune cells. CD4 cell count is a common indicator of immune function.

SIGNS AND SYMPTOMS OF HIV INFECTION

Depending on the stage of infection, the symptoms of HIV varies. Although those who have HIV are often most contagious in the first few months after becoming infected, many do not become aware of their condition until much later. Individuals may experience no symptoms in the first several weeks following first infection or flu-like symptoms, such as fever, headache, rash, or sore throat. They may also have other signs and symptoms including enlarged lymph nodes, weight loss, fever, diarrhea, and cough as the virus gradually weakens the immune system. In addition, they run the risk of contracting life-threatening conditions such as Kaposi's sarcoma and lymphomas, as well as cryptococcal meningitis, severe bacterial infections, and tuberculosis (TB).

MODE OF TRANSMISSION

Several bodily fluids from infected persons, including blood, breast milk, semen, and vaginal secretions, can transmit HIV from one person to the other. HIV can also be transmitted from an infected woman to her child when she is pregnant or during child birth. Normal daily contact, such as kissing, hugging, shaking hands, or sharing of personal items, food, or water, does not cause transmission of HIV infection in people. People with HIV who are on ART and have their viral load lowered; do not transfer the virus to their sexual partners significantly. Therefore, it is crucial to have early access to ART and assistance to stick with treatment in order to both improve the health of those who already have HIV and prevent HIV transmission.

PREVENTION OF PARENT TO CHILD TRANSMISSION

Out of 29 million annual pregnancies in India, 35,255 occur in HIV-positive pregnant women. Without any intervention, it is predicted that 10,361 infected newborns will be born each year.[5] It is a significant method of new HIV infections in children. About 4% of HIV infections in India are caused by parent-to-child transmission (PTCT). NACP is implementing the prevention of parent-to-child transmission (PPTCT) program to meet the objective of EMTCT.[6,7] The transmission of HIV to children born to women living with HIV may be averted in the majority of instances during pregnancy, labor, delivery, and breastfeeding when ART is provided to mothers and antiretroviral (ARV) prophylaxis is given to neonates. Of the anticipated 2,318,738 PLHIV in India in 2020, 81,430 are estimated to be children, which accounts for 3.5% of the total PLHIV cases.

All pregnant women have access to HIV diagnosis, preventive, care, and treatment services through the PPTCT programs.

Goals of PPTCT

- To prevent the transmission of HIV to children.
- Improve the survival and health of pregnant women, infants, and children in the context of HIV.

HIV transmission from mother to child occurs during pregnancy, delivery and breastfeeding. Major Factors that increase the risk of MTCT are listed in **Table 1**.

TABLE 1: Factors increasing MTCT.[6]

Factors during pregnancy	Factors during delivery	Factors while breastfeeding
• High viral load in the mother • A recent HIV infection while pregnant • Advanced disease in the mother • Viral, bacterial, and parasitic placental infection • Maternal malnutrition • STI	• New HIV infection • Advanced HIV disease/AIDS in mother • High viral load in mother • Prolonged labor • Premature rupture of membranes • Acute chorioamnionitis • Invasive delivery procedures • Premature baby • First infant in multiple birth	• New HIV infection during breastfeeding • Advanced HIV disease/AIDS in the mother • High maternal viral load • Duration of breastfeeding • Mixed feeding • Breast abscesses, nipple fissures, and mastitis • Maternal malnutrition • Oral disease in infant

(AIDS: acquired immunodeficiency syndrome; HIV: human immunodeficiency virus; MTCT: mother-to-child transmission; STI: sexually transmitted infection)
Source: Updated guidelines for Prevention of Parent to Child Transmission (PPTCT) of HIV using multi drug Anti-retroviral regimen in India December 2013.

TABLE 2: Risk of HIV transmission from mother to child with or without interventions.

ARV intervention	Risk of mother to child transmission of HIV
Not using ARV and breastfeeding	30–45%
Not using ARV, no breastfeeding	20–25%
Short course with one ARV and breastfeeding	15–25%
Short course with one ARV and no breastfeeding	5–15%
Short course with two ARV and breastfeeding	5%
3 ARV (ART) with breastfeeding	2%
3 ARV (ART) with no breastfeeding	1%

(ART: antiretroviral treatment; ARV: antiretroviral; HIV: human immunodeficiency virus)
Source:
1. National AIDS control Organisation & ICMR-National Institute of Medical Statistics (2021). India HIV Estimates 2020: Technical Brief. New Delhi: NACO, Ministry of Health and Family Welfare, Government of India.
2. World Health Organization. Antiretroviral drugs for treating pregnant women and preventing HIV infection in infants: towards universal access: recommendations for a public health approach–2006 version.

The risk of transmission depends on the periods of breastfeeding, maternal viral load, use of ART and exclusive or mixed feeding. The risk of HIV transmission from mother to child with or without interventions are listed in **Table 2**.

In order to prevent HIV transmission among women and children, the National PPTCT program acknowledges four essential components:[8]

Prong 1: HIV primary prevention, especially for women who are pregnant or planning a pregnancy

Prong 2: Preventing unplanned pregnancy in HIV-positive women

Prong 3: Prevention of HIV transmission from HIV-positive pregnant mothers to their unborn offspring

Prong 4: Provide care, support, and treatment to women living with HIV and to their children and families.

ANTENATAL CARE FOR HIV-POSITIVE PREGNANT WOMEN

- Counseling and HIV testing: All expectant mothers should get HIV education. Antenatal visits provide an opportunity for counseling regarding PPTCT.
- Choice of medical termination of pregnancy (MTP) and continuation of pregnancy
- Correction of anemia/diet supplements.
- Stop smoking/illicit drug abuse
- Regular structured antenatal care (ANC)
- Test/treat sexually transmitted infection/reproductive tract infection (STI/RTI), if any
- Early detection and management of opportunistic infection
- Timely ART initiation—tenofovir + lamivudine + dolutegravir (TLD)
- Hospital delivery
- Exclusive breastfeeding (EBF), early infant diagnosis (EID), cotrimoxazole preventive therapy (CPT), and 18 month testing.

In addition to standard tests and investigations, a specific emphasis should be placed on finding maternal health problems that might either directly or indirectly impair the fetus's health. Following special investigations are recommended to assess the infection and follow-up with treatment:

- Estimation of accurate gestational age
- *CD4 cell counts:* Done in the first visit and then every trimester during pregnancy
- *Viral load measurement:* At the time of the first appointment and between 32 and 36 weeks of pregnancy, it should be evaluated.
- *ART toxicity monitoring:* Before starting ART, complete blood count (CBC), blood urea nitrogen (BUN), creatinine and liver function test, and urinalysis should be done.
- *Gestational diabetes screening:* As the protease inhibitors tend to make HIV-infected people more susceptible to develop glucose intolerance, gestational diabetes mellitus (GDM) screening should be carried out earlier in HIV-positive pregnant women on ART regimens.
- *Viral hepatitis screening:* Both hepatitis B virus (HBV) and hepatitis C virus (HCV) have frequent coinfection with HIV.
- *TB testing:* In all patients with HIV, testing for TB is recommended.
- *STI screening:* All HIV-positive pregnant women need to be screened for syphilis, gonorrhea, *chlamydia,* and *Trichomonas* infection simultaneously. It has been shown that additional STIs are more frequently associated with stillbirth, low-birth-weight, premature preterm rupture of the membranes, and preterm delivery among HIV-positive women.
- Toxoplasma and CMV screening.
- *Vaccination assessment:* Pregnant HIV-positive women should take the pneumococcal and hepatitis A and B vaccinations in addition to the usual tetanus, diphtheria and acellular pertussis (Tdap) and influenza vaccines (if not prior vaccinated).
- *Behavioral counseling:* The couples should be counseled regarding avoidance of use of tobacco, alcohol, illicit drug, and also to avoid unprotected sexual intercourse.
- *Psychiatric evaluation:* Proper history regarding depression, anxiety, violence at home, and any such things must be addressed timely and properly.
- *Evaluation of opportunistic infection:* If CD4 count of HIV infected pregnant

women becomes <100/mL she should be given trimethoprim and sulfamethoxazole (TMP-SMX) for prevention of toxoplasmosis and *Pneumocystis carinii* infection.

INTERVENTIONS DURING LABOR AND DELIVERY

- Avoid unnecessary trauma during child birth
- Use noninvasive fetal monitoring
- Invasive procedures to be avoided
- Avoid routine episiotomy/support perineum
- Minimize the use of forceps or vacuum extractors
- After delivery of the head, infant's face should be wiped with gauze or cloth
- After delivery, the baby should be thoroughly wiped dry with a towel and then should be transferred to the mother.

Most of the mother to child transmission occurs during delivery. Hence adequate protection and care to the newborn should be given to reduce the risk of transmission, As per the national guidelines things to be done or not to be done are enlisted in **Table 3**.

Considerations in Mode of Delivery

Unless the mother has obstetrical grounds for a C-section, normal vaginal birth is recommended in India. Using ART can lower the risk of MTCT more effectively and safely than a C-section.

Safer Infant Feeding

The two infant feeding options available for the HIV-positive mother are EBF or exclusive replacement feeding (ERF). Counseling for infant feeding should begin in the antenatal period itself. EBF maximizes the chances of survival of these infants and is recommended as the preferred choice of infant feeding for HIV-exposed infants in India. Breastfeeding is made safe by giving ART to the mother and ARV prophylaxis to the baby. Mixed feeding increases the risk of transmission of HIV and should be avoided. The feeding option should be affordable, feasible, acceptable, sustainable, and safe (AFASS).

SAFER INFANT FEEDING (NATIONAL AIDS CONTROL ORGANISATION RECOMMENDATIONS)

- *EID–HIV positive:* These infants must be breastfed exclusively for the next 6 months. Up until 24 months, breastfeeding is allowed to continue.
- *EID–HIV negative:* Complementary feeding should be introduced after

TABLE 3: Immediate newborn care.[6]

Dos	Don'ts
Dry and warmth	Do not use mouth-operated suction
Clear airway	Do not do nasogastric tube suctioning in the newborn
Mouth and nostrils to be wiped as soon as head is delivered	
Cut cord with new blade in adequate light	
Initiate breastfeeding within 1 hour	
ARV prophylaxis to the baby as prescribed	

Source: Updated guidelines for Prevention of Parent to Child Transmission (PPTCT) of HIV using Multi Drug Antiretroviral Regimen in India December, 2013

6 months of EBF. Up to 24 months, breastfeeding should continue. When mothers decide to discontinue breastfeeding, they should do it gradually while taking the newborn and mother's comfort levels into account.
- A further HIV test is required. Accordance to the EID protocol, 6 weeks following the end of breastfeeding.

ANTIRETROVIRAL FOR THE MOTHER

Under the national program, it is recommended to provide lifelong ART for all pregnant and breastfeeding women living with HIV, where all pregnant women living with HIV receive a "fixed-dose combination (FDC)" triple-drug ART regimen regardless of CD4 count or clinical stage, both for their own health and to prevent vertical HIV transmission and for additional HIV prevention benefits. Currently, according to national recommendations, TLD is the optimal regimen for expectant mothers.[9] ART works for PPTCT by:
- Reduction of the maternal viral load
- Supplying the fetus with ARVs that stop the virus being transmitted from replicating
- Improving the mother's overall health
- Lowering the chance of transmission to the baby already exposed to HIV.

Goals of Antiretroviral Therapy

Human immunodeficiency virus (HIV) infection cannot be cured with ART because the ARV medications currently on the market cannot completely remove the virus from the body. Despite extended reduction of plasma viremia to undetectable levels by ART, HIV remains throughout the organs, tissues, and fluids (such as the brain, liver, and lymphoid tissue). The primary goals of ART are:
- Maximum and long-lasting reduction in plasma virus load
- Restoration of immunological systems
- Decreased transmission
- Reduction in new HIV infections.

Rationale for Transitioning to DTG-based Regimen

Currently recommended first-line ARV therapy is TLD (TDF + 3TC + DTG). It causes:
- Rapid viral load suppression (average 4 weeks for DTG vs. 12 weeks for EFV)
- Fewer toxicities and side effects
- Minimal discontinuations (<2%, less than with EFV)
- More potent regimen (no known treatment-emergent resistance across trials)
- Minimal drug interactions compared to other ARVs
- High genetic barrier
- Effective against HIV-2
- Harmonization across patient populations.

Dolutegravir

In 2013, the US Food and Drug Administration (FDA) granted it its initial approval for use. The World Health Organization (WHO) later recommended its use in 2019, and the National AIDS Control Organisation (NACO) Technical Resource Group approved its use starting in July 2020.[10] Dolutegravir is the recommended medication by NACO for the treatment of HIV-positive adults, adolescents, and children (over the age of 6 and weighing >20 kg) under the NACP. It is an "integrase inhibitor". It blocks the HIV integrase enzyme, which is essential for replication of the virus.

Antiretroviral Prophylaxis in Infant

Considering the likelihood of HIV transmission, the newborn is recommended to get ARV prophylaxis. Infants with low risk of HIV transmission should get single-drug

TABLE 4: Infant ARV prophylaxis.[8,11]

HIV risk status	Option for ARV prophylaxis	Breastfeeding	Duration of ARV
Low-risk infants: • Infants born to mothers with suppressed viral load	Syrup nevirapine (NVP) or syrup zidovudine	EBF ERF	6 weeks regardless of feeding option

High-risk infants:
• Infants born to HIV-positive mother not on ART
• Maternal viral load not done after 32 weeks of pregnancy till delivery
• Maternal viral load not suppressed between 32 weeks of pregnancy till delivery
• Mother newly identified HIV-positive within 6 weeks of delivery
	• Options for dual prophylaxis: Syrup NVP + syrup zidovudine
	• Duration of dual ARV prophylaxis:
	  – In case of ERF: From birth till 6 weeks of age
	  – In case of EBF: From birth till 12 weeks of age
		EBF
		
		ERF
			12 weeks
			
			6 weeks

(ARV: antiretroviral; EBF: exclusive breastfeeding; ERF: exclusive replacement feeding; HIV: human immunodeficiency virus)
Source: National guidelines for HIV care and treatment 2021.

ARV prophylaxis for 6 weeks (regardless of type of feeding). Dual-drug ARV prophylaxis is advised in infants with high risk for HIV transmission, the recommended period varies depending on the method of feeding (for 6 weeks if using replacement feeding and 12 weeks if using breastfeeding).[8] Details of the Antiretroviral therapy to be offered to newborn are listed in **Table 4**.

GOALS AND TARGETS OF NACP AND EMTCT

An uniform "National Guidelines on HIV Care and Treatment" remain the cornerstone for standardizing treatment strategies and consequently improving the quality of HIV care across all sectors of healthcare in order to accomplish the sustainable development growth (SDG) objective of "end of AIDS as a public health threat" by 2030. India is committed to achieve the "EMTCT HIV objective" of keeping women alive and preventing the birth of any children with HIV. UNAIDS has set the target of 95-95-95 by the year 2030. The following targets for process indicators are required for EMTCT validation and must be maintained for at least 2 years:

- First 95 implies that 95% of estimated people living with HIV to be diagnosed
- Second 95% is out of the identified cases 95% to be connected to ART services
- Third 95% implies in 95% of PLHIV those who are on ART the viral load should be suppressed which is possible with continuous ART drug adherence.

REFERENCES

1. National Aids Control Organization, Ministry of Health and Family Welfare, Government of India: Annual report 2018-2019.
2. UNAIDS. (2021). Global AIDS update-2021: Confronting inequalities. [online] Available from: https://www.unaids.org/sites/default/files/media_asset/2021-global-aids-update_en.pelf. [Last accessed April, 2023].
3. National AIDS Control Organisation; ICMR-National Institute of Medical Statistics. India HIV Estimates 2020: Technical Brief. New Delhi: NACO, Minisuy of Health and Family Welfare, Government of India; 2021.

4. HIV.gov. (2023). What Are HIV and AIDS? [online] Available from: https://www.hiv.gov/hiv-basics/overview/a bout-hiv-and-aids/what-are-hiv-and-aids. [Last accessed April, 2023].
5. National AIDS control organization: Technical estimate report (20 15)
6. NACO. (2013). Updated Guidelines for Prevention of Parent to Child Transmission (PPTCT) of HIV using Multi Drug Antiretroviral Regimen in India. [online] Available from: http://naco.gov.in/sites/default/files/National_Guidelines_for_PPTCT.pdf. [Last accessed April, 2023].
7. National guidelines for HIV care and treatment 2021: Mother to Child Transmission. NACEP. National AIDS Clinical Expert Panel. NACO. National AIDS Control Organization.
8. Strategy Document: National AIDS and STD Control Programme Phase-V. (2021-26). New Delhi: NACO, Ministry of Health and Family Welfare, Government of India.
9. National AIDS Control Organization. NACO (2021).
10. World Health Organization. Updated recommendations on first-line and second-line antiretroviral regimes and post-exposure prophylaxis and recommendations on early infant diagnosis of HIV. Geneva, Switzerland: World Health Organization; 2018.
11. World Health Organization. Antiretroviral drugs for treating pregnant women and preventing HIV infection in infants: towards universal access: recommendations for a public health approach, 2006 version. Geneva, Switzerland: World Health Organization; 2006.

17

SARS-CoV-2 during Pregnancy

Sudesh Agrawal

■ INTRODUCTION

Severe acute respiratory syndrome coronavirus 2 (SARS-CoV-2) is a novel, enveloped single stranded ribonucleic acid (RNA) coronavirus. Other names are coronavirus disease-2019 (COVID-19) and coronavirus. First case of SARS-CoV-2 was detected in Wuhan, China in December, 2019. The World Health Organization (WHO) has declared it pandemic on 11 March, 2020.[1] Many variants of this virus have been identified since the diagnosis of the first case.

The SARS-CoV-2 virus can be transmitted by human-to-human via droplets, aerosols, close person-to-person contact, and direct contact with fomites. The virus enters the body via the nasal passage and infects pulmonary cells via the angiotensin-converting enzyme 2 (ACE2) receptors and uses transmembrane serine protease 2 (TMPRSS2) for S protein priming.[2-4] This is followed by viral replication and release of the virus causing pyroptosis (inflammation-mediated programmed cell death occurring in response to a pathological stimulus of the host cell). This releases adenosine triphosphate (ATP) and nucleic acids, also known as damage-associated molecular patterns (DAMPs), that trigger an inflammatory response from neighboring cells.[5]

▌ PREGNANT WOMEN AND "FETUS" ARE AT HIGH RISK

Pregnancy is associated with many adaptive changes in physiology and immune system and this makes pregnant women and their fetuses "at high risk".

During pregnancy chest wall compliance and functional residual capacity (FRC) decreases by 35–40%, with compensatory respiratory alkalemia.[6,7] The oxygen dissociation curve is shifted to the right, which is beneficial to oxygen transfer across the placenta, thus making more oxygen available to the fetus.[8] This altered respiratory state can decompensate rapidly in presence of pulmonary complications.[9]

Pregnancy is a state of altered immunological response to allow for the growth of semi allogeneic fetus. There is a proinflammatory stage at the time of implantation and placentation in the first trimester, anti-inflammatory stage during growth of the fetus and again a proinflammatory stage during initiation of parturition.[10] Adaptive immune responses during most of the pregnancy are down regulated and number of T and B, monocytes, and circulating natural killer (NK) cells are decreased.[11] $CD4^+$ (T-cell population) shifts toward the Th2 phenotype over Th1 phenotype. Progesterone has immunomodulatory properties. Under the influence of hormones, mucous membrane of upper respiratory tract (nose, pharynx, and trachea) has thickening, mild hyperemia, edema, and is prone to upper respiratory tract infection.

Pulmonary endothelial cell dysfunction plays an important role in the onset and progression of acute respiratory distress syndrome (ARDS).

Analysis of available data indicates that Hispanic or Black pregnant women are disproportionately affected by SARS-CoV-2 infection. This disparity is related to social determinants of health, current and historic inequities in access to healthcare/other resources, and structural racism.

■ PRESENTATION OF SARS-COV-2

Patient can remain asymptomatic or have mild symptoms in form of fever, cough, and myalgia/fatigue (main symptoms) or loss of taste and smell, abdominal pain, etc., as in nonpregnant individuals. Symptoms may appear 2–14 days after exposure to the virus. In a few cases, life-threatening pneumonia infection/ARDS can be caused by coronaviruses. Severe illness includes illness that may require admission to an intensive care unit (ICU), invasive ventilation, extracorporeal membrane oxygenation (ECMO) or which may culminate in death.

As compared to nonpregnant patients infected with COVID-19, pregnant patients with similar infection are more likely to get severe illness and bad outcome. After adjustments have been made for age, race/ethnicity, and underlying medical conditions, pregnant women have significantly:

- Higher rates of ICU admission [10.5 vs. 3.9 cases per 1,000 cases; adjusted risk ratio (aRR) 3.0; 95% confidence interval (CI), 2.6–3.4]
- Mechanical ventilation (MV) (2.9 vs. 1.1 cases per 1,000 cases; aRR 2.9; 95% CI, 2.2–3.8)
- ECMO (0.7 vs. 0.3 cases per 1,000 cases; aRR 2.4; 95% CI, 1.5–4.0), and death (1.5 corona positive vs. 1.2 cases per 1,000 cases; aRR 1.7; 95% CI, 1.2–2.4).[12]

The Centers for Disease Control and Prevention (CDC) analysis compared cases in pregnant women versus nonpregnant women aged 15–44 years reported from 01/01/2020 to 25/12/2021. Results indicated bad outcome for the pregnant women.

- There was five times the risk of admission to an ICU
- 76% increased risk of invasive ventilation or ECMO
- There was further worsened outcome with Delta variant, which emerged in June, 2021. Data published in June, 2022,[13] have found that, when comparing pregnant women aged 15–44 years in the pre-Delta period (01/01/2020–26/06/2021) with those in the Delta period (27/06/2021–25/12/2021) outcome during pregnancy was worse.
- During Delta period the risk of admission in the ICU was 41% higher.
- During Delta period the risk of invasive ventilation or ECMO was 83% higher.
- During Delta period the risk of death was 3.3 times the risk in the pre-Delta period.

■ EFFECT OF SARS-COV-2 INFECTION ON PERINATAL OUTCOME

Any ongoing proinflammatory signal in the early pregnancy can lead to miscarriage and preterm birth if in later pregnancy (before term).

Results of the Gestational Research Assessments for COVID-19 (GRAVID)[14] study show that pregnant patients who had SARS-CoV-2 infection prior to 28 weeks of gestation had a subsequent:

- Increased risk of fetal/neonatal death (aRR 1.97; 95% CI, 1.01–3.85),
- Preterm birth at <37 weeks (aRR 1.29; 95% CI, 1.02–1.63),
- Hypertensive disorders of pregnancy (aRR 1.74; 95% CI, 1.19–2.55).

Adverse perinatal outcomes were more common in patients with severe or critical disease than in asymptomatic patients with SARS-CoV-2 infection,[15] including:
- Increased incidence of cesarean delivery (59.6% vs. 34.0% of patients; aRR 1.57; 95% CI, 1.30–1.90),
- Hypertensive disorders of pregnancy (40.4% vs. 18.8%; aRR 1.61; 95% CI, 1.18–2.20),
- Preterm birth (41.8% vs. 11.9%; aRR 3.53; 95% CI, 2.42–5.14).

RISK OF VERTICAL OR MOTHER-TO-CHILD TRANSMISSION OF SARS-COV-2 INFECTION DURING PREGNANCY

- Analysis of the available data shows that most infants borne to SARS-CoV-2 infected mothers are negative (for SARS-CoV-2 test) at birth.
- Some newborns who are positive for COVID-19 shortly after birth.[16] We however, do not know if these newborns were affected before, during, or after birth.
- Soon after birth, newborn blood was found positive for Immunoglobulin M (IgM) antibodies against SARS-CoV-2 infection.[17,18] Advanced electron microscopy pictures have confirmed presence of COVID-19 virus like particles in the placenta.[19,20] These findings indicate possible vertical transmission of the infection.
- Transplacental transmission is expected to be hematogenous. In these cases, nasopharyngeal swab may be negative for the virus.
- Role of immunoglobulin G (IgG) antibodies and passive protection remains to be elucidated.
- Most of the newborns, even if positive at birth, remain asymptomatic or have mild illness that recovers well. Only a few reports have reported severe illness/death in the newborns.
- Further studies are needed.

PREVENTION OF SARS-COV-2 INFECTION DURING PREGNANCY

Prevention is Better than Cure—General Measures

Pregnant or lactating women (especially in presence of comorbidities) should:
- Avoid crowded indoor places/contact with COVID-19 infected individuals
- Should maintain a distance of 6 feet at all times (social distancing)
- Should wear well-fitting face mask properly (should avoid the mask with expirator, if infected)
- Should avoid touching fomites. They should wash their hands frequently with soap and water or with disinfectant (containing 60% alcohol)
- Should consult health facility, even if minimal symptoms.

PREGNANCY AND VACCINATION AGAINST SARS-COV-2

- Pregnant people should be counseled about the benefits of COVID-19 vaccination, which include a decreased risk of severe disease and hospitalization for the pregnant person and a decreased risk of hospitalization for the infant in the first 6 months of life. All eligible persons, including pregnant and lactating individuals and those who are planning to become pregnant should receive

COVID-19 vaccine (full course of two doses and/or booster dose), COVID-19 vaccines can be administered regardless of trimester and in concert with other vaccines that are recommended during pregnancy.[21] Reported side effects are local injection site pain, nausea, and vomiting as are reported in nonpregnant women.
- The available data indicate that vaccine derived antibodies are passively transferred to the neonate during pregnancy and lactation.
- People who previously received monoclonal antibodies (mAbs) as part of COVID-19 treatment, postexposure prophylaxis, or preexposure prophylaxis can be vaccinated at any time; COVID-19 vaccination no longer needs to be delayed following receipt of mAbs.[22]
- Vaccines are being made available in India after registration at the COVID-19 Vaccine Intelligence Network (CoWIN) platform or using the Aarogya Setu application. The vaccines are made available free of cost at most of the places. At private clinics they may be chargeable.
- Mainly Covishield and Covaxin are being distributed in India and are being used in pregnant women.

Covishield

This vaccine was developed by Oxford-AstraZeneca and manufactured in India by the Serum Institute of India. The Covishield is made from modified and weakened adenovirus (a common cold virus) taken from chimpanzees. It is administered in two doses between 4 and 12 weeks apart. It has an efficacy of 76% after the first dose, and 81.3% after the second dose. Common side effects include headache, fatigue, muscle or joint pain, fever, chills, and nausea.

Covaxin (BBV152)

The Covaxin vaccine was developed by Bharat Biotech in collaboration with the Indian Council of Medical Research (ICMR) and India's National Institute of Virology. It is made using inactivated coronaviruses that are safe to be injected into patients. It is given in two doses, 4 weeks apart. It has an efficacy rate of 81%. Possible side effects include pain, swelling, itching, fever, rashes, overall weakness, nausea, vomiting, and in rare cases, difficulty in breathing and swelling of the throat and face.

Sputnik V was approved by the Government as a third vaccine.

PRE- AND POSTEXPOSURE PROPHYLAXIS WITH SARS-COV-2 MONOCLONAL ANTIBODIES

Pre- and postexposure prophylaxis with SARS-CoV-2 mAbs may be considered in pregnant and lactating females. Postexposure prophylaxis is given to women, who have been exposed to SARS-CoV-2. These individuals include those who have had a recent exposure to an individual with SARS-CoV-2 for a cumulative total of 15 minutes or more over a 24-hour period or there is a recent occurrence of SARS-CoV-2 infection in other individuals in the same institutional setting and:
- She is not fully vaccinated
- She is unable to mount adequate immune response to vaccination
- She cannot be vaccinated due to potential for severe or life-threatening reaction to vaccine or its components.

The authorized anti-SARS-CoV-2 mAbs are IgG antibodies and are expected to cross the placenta.

Lactating women with one or more risk factors for severe COVID-19 illness may receive mAbs for treatment or postexposure prophylaxis. There is no need to temporarily discontinue breastfeeding when receiving mAbs.

MANAGEMENT OF PATIENTS WITH SARS-COV-2 INFECTION

There should be shared decision making between patients and providers. asymptomatic women or in presence of mild symptoms can have domiciliary care with isolation and proper support system. Social support and counseling are important.

Pregnancy is a risk factor for severe disease. Obstetric care clinicians may consider the use of mAbs for the treatment of outpatient COVID-19 positive pregnant individuals with mild-to-moderate symptoms, particularly if one or more additional risk factors are present [e.g., body mass index (BMI) >25, chronic kidney disease, diabetes mellitus, and cardiovascular disease).

Routine antenatal care must be continued. Tele medicine/telehealth may be used, if feasible.

Considering bad outcome in severely ill patients, threshold for hospitalization/ICU care should be lowered and treatment should be started early. Risk versus benefit should be carefully considered and no female should be denied treatment, on the grounds of pregnancy or lactation. The illness severity, underlying comorbidities, and the clinical status of the patient should be considered, to assess potential hospitalization.

- The facilities, where pregnant patients with SARS-CoV-2 infection can be admitted should be fully equipped and manned.
- There must be facilities for monitoring of fetal well-being, fetal heart rate, and uterine contractions in suitable cases
- The delivery planning should be individualized.
- A multispeciality, team-based approach should be followed. Team may include obstetric, pediatric, maternal-fetal medicine, infectious disease, and pulmonary critical care specialists, as appropriate.

Timing and Mode of Delivery

- There is insufficient data available because of the novelty of the virus and noninclusion of pregnant and lactating females, in most of the trials.
- In asymptomatic or mild cases timing and mode of delivery has to be decided according to obstetric indications.
- In patients, who had SARS CoV-2 infection early in pregnancy, timing and mode of delivery has to be decided according to obstetric indications.
- In cases of severe SARS CoV-2, especially if the mother is in ICU in moribund condition or is on ECMO support, maternal welfare takes priority.
- Therapeutic management of SARS-CoV-2 infection during pregnancy remains largely the same as in the nonpregnant patients (level AIII evidence).
- Some drugs like molnupiravir should be used only if absolutely necessary and no suitable alternative is available.
- There is insufficient data for use of anticoagulants in pregnant patients with SARS-CoV-2 infection without venous thromboembolism. There remains a risk of bleeding and increased complications.
- Antenatal steroid use for threatened preterm labor is likely to be safe and in severe maternal disease also steroid may be administered.
- Respectful maternity care should be ensured. Companion may be permitted during labor, provided they are trained to use personal protective equipment (PPE) and take all the precautions necessary for infection control.

CONSIDERATION OF COMORBIDITY AND OTHER PREGNANCY COMPLICATIONS IN SARS-COV-2 INFECTED WOMEN

Pregnancies affected by preeclampsia have significant endothelial dysfunction and uteroplacental blood flow may be already compromised. These women are at a particular risk of development of COVID-19 complication with multiple organ failure with severe outcome. In these cases, diagnosis and treatment becomes challenging.

Use of Anticoagulants during Pregnancy

Pregnancy is a hypercoagulable state. Pregnant and postpartum women have four- to fivefold increased risk of thromboembolism. COVID-19 infection also leads to coagulopathy. Pregnant patients hospitalized for severe COVID-19 are given prophylactic anticoagulants, unless contraindicated. During pregnancy, there are higher levels of circulating coagulation and fibrinolytic factors, such as plasmin, and these may be implicated in the pathogenesis of SARS-CoV-2 infection.

Contraindications for the use of therapeutic anticoagulation in patients with COVID-19 include a platelet count $<50 \times 10^9$/L, hemoglobin (Hb) <8 g/dL, the need for dual antiplatelet therapy, bleeding within the past 30 days that required hospitalization, a history of a bleeding disorder, or an inherited or active acquired bleeding disorder

Molnupiravir and pregnancy (Level AIII Evidence)

- Animal studies have reported fetal toxicities of the molnupiravir. However, if benefit outweighs the risk or if other therapy is not available, molnupiravir may be used, after proper counseling of the patient. Period of embryogenesis (up to 10 weeks) should be avoided.
- No data is available for use of molnupiravir in lactating mothers. The Food and Drug Administration Emergency Use Authorization for molnupiravir states that lactating people should not breastfeed their infants during treatment with molnupiravir and for 4 days after the final dose.
- Breast milk should be expressed and discarded during molnupiravir use.

Use of antivirals (including antibody products), immunomodulators, and other medications during pregnancy with SARS-CoV-2 infection **Table 1**.

Obstetric care clinicians should be aware that the concomitant use of Paxlovid and certain other drugs (including medications used in obstetric settings such as nifedipine, methylergonovine, fentanyl, midazolam, or betamethasone) may result in potentially significant drug interactions.

If tranexamic acid is required for control of postpartum hemorrhage, one must consider hypercoagulable state of pregnancy added on to the thrombotic risk of COVID-19 infection.

SARS COV-2 INFECTION AND BREAST FEEDING

- The majority of the studies have not found SARS-CoV-2 in breast milk.
- Therefore, breastfeeding is not contraindicated in presence of suspected or confirmed SARS-CoV-2 infection, provided mother is healthy enough to take care of the baby.
- Baby may be roomed in with the mother, keeping a distance of 6 feet (and a physical partition, if possible) from the mother in positive case.

TABLE 1: Therapeutic management of hospitalized adults with COVID-19[23]			
Severity of the disease	**Clinical Scenario**	**Recommendations**	**Remarks**
Hospitalized for indications other than COVID-19	Mild/moderate disease	Treatment same as in non-hospitalized women	
Hospitalized but does not require oxygen supplementation	All patients	No need of dexamethasone/systemic corticosteroid (AIIa)	Use steroids only if indicated for obstetric condition
If at high risk		Use remdesivir (BIII)	
Hospitalized and require oxygen (Conventional)	• If only minimal support of oxygen is required • Most patients • Patients who are on already dexamethasone and are deteriorating or need increasing oxygen and with systemic signs of inflammation	• Use remdesivir (BIIa) • Use dexamethasone plus remdesivir (BIIa). If remdesivir cannot be obtained, use dexamethasone (BI) • Add IV tocilizumab or oral baricitinib (BIIa)	
Hospitalized and require HFNC oxygen or NIV	Most patients	Promptly start one of the following: • Dexamethasone plus oral baricitinib (AI) • Dexamethasone plus IV tocilizumab (BIIa) • If baricitinib, tofacitinib, tocilizumab or sarilumab are not available; use dexamethasone* (AI)	Add Remdesivir to any of these options in certain patients (CIIa)
Hospitalized and require MV or ECMO	Most patients	Promptly start one of the following: • Dexamethasone plus oral baricitinib (BIIa) • Dexamethasone plus IV tocilizumab (BIIa) • If baricitinib, tofacitinib, tocilizumab or sarilumab are not available; use dexamethasone* (AI)	

(CDC: Centers for Disease Control and Prevention; COVID-19: coronavirus disease-2019; ECMO: extracorporeal membrane oxygenation; ED: emergency department; HFNC: high-flow nasal cannula; Hb: hemoglobin; ICU: intensive care unit; IL: interleukin; IV: intravenous; JAK: Janus kinase; mAb: monoclonal antibody; MV: mechanical ventilation; NIV: noninvasive ventilation; the Panel: the COVID-19 Treatment Guidelines Panel.)

*If a Janus kinase (JAK) inhibitor or an anti-IL-6 receptor mAb is not readily available, start dexamethasone while waiting for the additional immunomodulator to be acquired. If neither of the other immunomodulators can be obtained, use dexamethasone alone. Clinicians may consider adding remdesivir to 1 of the recommended immunomodulator combinations in patients who require HFNC oxygen or NIV, including immunocompromised patients. The Panel recommends against the use of remdesivir without immunomodulators in these patients (AIIa).

Contd...

Contd…

Note:
- Evidence suggests that the benefit of remdesivir is greatest when the drug is given early in the course of COVID-19 (e.g., within 10 days of symptom onset).
- Corticosteroids that are prescribed for an underlying condition should be continued.
- The use of anticoagulants needs to be individualized, as there is a risk of bleeding, especially after an operative delivery.
- Contraindications for the use of therapeutic anticoagulation in patients with COVID-19 include a platelet count 50×10^9/L, Hb 8 g/dL, the need for dual antiplatelet therapy, bleeding within the past 30 days that required an Emergency visit or hospitalization, a history of a bleeding disorder, or an inherited or active acquired bleeding disorder.

Source: These recommendations are based on NIH. (2022). COVID-19 Treatment Guidelines. Available from: https://files.covid19treatment guidelines.nih.gov/guidelines/archive/covid19treatmentguidelines-08-08-2022.pdf.

- Mother has to follow the precautions like washing the hands with soap and water/antiseptic solution with 60% alcohol, before and after handling the baby. Breasts and nipple must be cleaned each time, before and after feed.
- Must wear properly fitting facemask and consistently all the time.
- Brest pump must be thoroughly cleaned, in case expressed breast milk is used.

POSTPARTUM PATIENT AND SARS-COV-2 INFECTION

Essential management of postpartum patient remains same as in the nonpregnant patients.

POINTS TO REMEMBER

- Most of the women affected with SARS-CoV-2 infection remain asymptomatic or have mild disease and can be managed as outdoor patients.
- Risk of hospitalization, ICU care, invasive ventilation, ECMO support, and even death in pregnant women affected with COVID-19 are more as compared to nonpregnant women affected similarly. In presence of comorbidities, risk further increases.
- Adverse perinatal outcome in form of preterm delivery and even death is more common in patients with severe disease as compared to asymptomatic women.
- Prevention is better. Social distancing, well-fitting mask, and hand hygiene are essential. Full course of vaccine with booster should be taken by all women who are pregnant or are planning to become pregnant.
- Pregnant patients with COVID-19 should be delivered in well-equipped and managed units where specialist care is available.
- Shared decision making and counseling is very important.
- SARS-CoV-2 positive women can directly breastfeed the baby, provided they follow hand hygiene, cough etiquette, proper mask, and cleaning of breast/nipple/breast pump properly.
- Care should be taken of the mental health of the patient. Respectful maternity experience and positive parturition experience should be the aim.

REFERENCES

1. https://www.euro.who.int/en/health-topics/health-emergencies/coronavirus-covid-19/news/news/2020/3/who-announces-covid-19-outbreak-a-pandemic.

2. Cascella M, Rajnik M, Cuomo A, Dulebohn SC, Di Napoli R. Features, Evaluation and Treatment Coronavirus (COVID-19) (Online). https://www.ncbi.nlm.nih.gov/pubmed/32150360.
3. Heurich A, Hofmann-Winkler H, Gierer S, Liepold T, Jahn O, Pohlmann S. TMPRSS2 and ADAM17 Cleave ACE2 Differentially and Only Proteolysis by TMPRSS2 Augments Entry Driven by the Severe Acute Respiratory Syndrome Coronavirus Spike Protein. J. Virol. 2014;88:1293–1307. doi: 10.1128/JVI.02202-13.
4. Tay MZ, Poh CM, Rénia L, MacAry PA, Ng LFP. The trinity of COVID-19: immunity, inflammation and intervention. Nat Rev Immunol 20: 363–374, 2020. doi:10.1038/s41577-020-0311-8.
5. Rabi FA, Al Zoubi MS, Kasasbeh GA, Salameh DM, Al-Nasser AD. SARS-CoV-2 and coronavirus disease 2019: what we know so far. Pathogens 9: 231, 2020. doi:10.3390/pathogens9030231.
6. Marx GF, Murthy PK, Orkin LR Static compliance before and after vaginal delivery. Br J Anaesth. 1970;42(12):1100–1104. doi: 10.1093/bja/42.12.1100.
7. Hegewald MJ, Crapo RO. Respiratory physiology in pregnancy. Clin Chest Med. 2011;32(1):1–13. doi: 10.1016/j.ccm.2010.11.001.
8. Wise RA, Polito AJ, Krishnan V. Respiratory physiologic changes in pregnancy. Immunol Allergy Clin N Am. 2006;26(1):1–12. doi: 10.1016/j.iac.2005.10.004.
9. Jensen D, Wolfe LA, Slatkovska L. Effects of human pregnancy on the ventilator chemoreflex response to carbon dioxide. Am J Physiol Regul Integr Comp Physiol. 2005;288(5):R1369–R1375. doi: 10.1152/ajpregu.00862.2004.
10. Mor G, Cardenas I, Abrahams V, Guller S. Inflammation and pregnancy: the role of the immune system at the implantation site. Ann N Y Acad Sci. 2011;1221(1):80–87. doi: 1111/j.1749-6632.2010.05938.x.
11. Aghaeepour N, Ganio EA, Mcilwain D. An immune clock of human pregnancy. Sci Immunol. 2017;2(15):eaan2946. doi: 10.1126/sciimmunol.aan2946.
12. Zambrano LD, Ellington S, Strid P, et al. Update: characteristics of symptomatic women of reproductive age with laboratory-confirmed SARS-CoV-2 infection by pregnancy status—United States, January 22–October 3, 2020. MMWR Morb Mortal Wkly Rep. 2020;69(44):1641-1647. Available at: https://www.ncbi.nlm.nih.gov/pubmed/33151921.
13. Penelope Strid and others, Coronavirus Disease 2019 (COVID-19) Severity Among Women of Reproductive Age With Symptomatic Laboratory-Confirmed Severe Acute Respiratory Syndrome Coronavirus 2 (SARS-CoV-2) Infection by Pregnancy Status—United States, 1 January 2020–25 December 2021, Clinical Infectious Diseases, Volume 75, Issue Supplement_2, 1 October 2022, Pages S317–S325, https://doi.org/10.1093/cid/ciac479.
14. Hughes BL, Sandoval GJ, Metz TD, et al. First- or second-trimester SARS-CoV-2 infection and subsequent pregnancy outcomes. Am J Obstet Gynecol. 2023;228(2):226.e221-226.e229. Available at: https://www.ncbi.nlm.nih.gov/pubmed/35970201.
15. Metz TD, Clifton RG, Hughes BL, et al. Disease severity and perinatal outcomes of pregnant patients with coronavirus disease 2019 (COVID-19). Obstet Gynecol. 2021;137(4):571-580. Available at: https://www.ncbi.nlm.nih.gov/pubmed/33560778.
16. Kirtsman M, Diambomba Y, Poutanen SM, et al. Probable congenital SARS-CoV-2 infection in a neonate born to a woman with active SARS-CoV-2 infection. CMAJ. 2020;192:E647–E650.
17. Zeng H, Xu C, Fan J, et al. Antibodies in infants born to mothers with COVID-19 pneumonia. JAMA. 2020;323:1848–1849.
18. Dong L, Tian J, He S, et al. Possible vertical transmission of SARS-CoV-2 from an infected mother to her newborn. JAMA. 2020;323:1846–1848.
19. Patanè L, Morotti D, Giunta MR, et al. Vertical transmission of COVID-19: SARSCoV-2 RNA on the fetal side of the placenta in

pregnancies with COVID-19 positive mothers and neonates at birth. Am J Obstet Gynecol MFM. 2020.
20. Algarroba GN, Rekawek P, Vahanian SA, et al. Visualization of severe acute respiratory syndrome coronavirus 2 invading the human placenta using electron microscopy. Am J Obstet Gynecol. 2020;223:275–278.
21. CDC. (2023). Summary Document for Interim Clinical Considerations for Use of COVID-19 Vaccines Currently Authorized or Approved in the United States. [online] Available from: https://www.cdc.gov/vaccines/covid-19/downloads/summary-interim- clinical - considerations.pdf.
22. Society for Maternal-Fetal Medicine. Provider considerations for engaging in COVID-19 vaccine counseling with pregnant and lactating patients. 2022. Available at: https://www.smfm.org/covidclinical.
23. COVID-19 Treatment Guidelines Panel. Coronavirus Disease 2019 (COVID-19) Treatment Guidelines. National Institutes of Health. Available at https://www.euro.who.int/en/health-topics/health-emergencies/coronavirus-covid-19/news/news/2020/3/who-announces-covid-19-outbreak-a-pandemic Cascella M, Rajnik M, Cuomo A, Dulebohn SC, Di Napoli R. Features, Evaluation and Treatment.

CHAPTER 18

Pregnancy-related Constipation

Saket Kumar, Lakshit Tomar, Vijay Prakash Singh

■ INTRODUCTION

Constipation is one of the most common gastrointestinal problems experienced during pregnancy, affecting between 11 and 31% of expectant mothers.[1] Women without prior history of bowel problems may experience de novo constipation during pregnancy and in addition, women with preexisting constipation may experience worsening of their symptoms during pregnancy.[2] Pregnant women are susceptible to developing constipation due to various physiological and anatomical changes in the gastrointestinal tract.

While constipation during pregnancy is often labeled as usual or even considered "physiologic" in obstetric textbooks, information on bowel dysfunction during pregnancy is limited.[3] The majority of research on pregnancy-related constipation is constrained by retrospective study designs and inconsistent or inadequately defined definitions of constipation.[4,5] The Rome IV criteria **(Box 1)**, designed to define chronic constipation in the general population, are applied to pregnant women as well.[6]

A simplified criteria for diagnosing constipation includes a low frequency of stools (less than three per week), passage of hard stools, and/or difficulties with the evacuation of stool **(Box 2)**. These criteria are easier to use in routine clinical practice and are reliable indicators of constipation in pregnant women.[2]

BOX 1: Rome IV criteria for chronic constipation.

Diagnostic criteria: Must include two or more of the following occurring at least once per week for a minimum of 1 month with insufficient criteria for a diagnosis of irritable bowel syndrome (IBS):
1. Straining during >25% of defecations
2. Lumpy or hard stools (the Bristol Stool Form Scale 1–2) >25% of defecations
3. Sensation of incomplete evacuation >25% of defecations
4. Sensations of anorectal obstruction/blockage >25% of defecations
5. Manual maneuvers to facilitate >25% of defecations (e.g., digital evacuation)
6. Fewer than three spontaneous bowel movements per week

BOX 2: Simplified diagnostic criteria for constipation during pregnancy.

- Infrequent passage of stool (less than three times per week)
- Passage of hard, dry stools
- Difficult evacuation

■ SYMPTOMATOLOGY

A prospective study showed that constipation most commonly occurs in the first two trimesters of pregnancy. The prevalence of functional constipation in the first and second trimesters varies between 35 and 39%, and is 21% in the third trimester.[7]

Women commonly report the passage of dry, hard stools accompanied by pain and straining. Some women may present with a distressing sensation of incomplete evacuation, and in extreme instances, they may even necessitate digital fecal evacuation. Fecal impaction and straining may lead to urinary retention and rectal prolapse in rare instances. It is important to document any history of laxative or enema use, including the dosage and frequency of treatment. For patients experiencing per rectal bleeding or exhibiting associated features of bowel obstruction, evaluation by a colorectal surgeon or gastroenterologist is recommended.[8]

PATHOPHYSIOLOGY

The exact cause of this troubling problem remains unknown, and it is likely to be multifactorial **(Box 3)**. Elevated progesterone hormone level, causing decreased smooth muscle contractility and slow gastrointestinal transit, is frequently implicated. Additionally, reduced motilin levels during pregnancy have also been described as cause for constipation.[9,10] Several other factors have been identified as potential contributors to the development of constipation during pregnancy. These include the mechanical impact of the gravid uterus and the supplementation of dietary vitamins. Pregnant women may experience constipation for reasons similar to nonpregnant women, such as metabolic abnormalities (e.g., hypothyroidism) or the use of constipating medications (e.g., calcium or iron supplements). Constipation during pregnancy may be rarely attributed to structural abnormalities such as colonic strictures, painful anal fissures, or thrombosed piles.[11]

■ EVALUATION

Constipation related to pregnancy does not require an extensive evaluation, and most patients respond to simple measures such as dietary changes and laxatives. The approach to constipation in pregnancy is similar to that used for the general population, with particular emphasis on ensuring the safety of medications used during pregnancy.[5] Diagnostic investigations are conducted to exclude treatable disorders like hypothyroidism or hypercalcemia. Women experiencing worsening symptoms, per anal bleeding and progressive abdominal distention, should undergo further evaluation by a specialist gastroenterologist.[8] When indicated, digital rectal examination and lower gastrointestinal endoscopy are performed. Ultrasound and magnetic resonance imaging (MRI) are imaging modality of choice during pregnancy as they lack ionizing radiation.

■ TREATMENT

Dietary Modification and Exercise

Most pregnancy-related constipation can be successfully treated by promoting a diet high in fiber and increasing fluid intake. Incorporating fiber into the diet through a wheat- or corn-based fiber supplement has been shown to increase stool frequency and enhance stool form in pregnant women with

---

BOX 3: Causes of constipation in pregnancy.

- Dehydration (anorexia, nausea/vomiting, low fluid intake)
- Hormonal (progesterone, hypothyroidism, reduced motilin levels)
- Mechanical (gravid uterus)
- Drugs (iron, tocolytics, calcium)
- Preexisting constipation
- Low fiber intake
- Irritable bowel syndrome
- *Mechanical causes:* Colonic stricture, bands, acute anal fissure, thrombosed hemorrhoids

constipation, as demonstrated in a 2-week placebo-controlled trial.[12] The suggested daily intake of dietary fiber is typically in the range of 20–35 grams. The laxation effect of fiber may take 3–7 days to become apparent. It is noteworthy that consuming large quantities of fiber too rapidly can lead to abdominal bloating, gaseous distention, cramping, and diarrhea. To mitigate these effects, it is advisable to ensure adequate fluid intake when consuming fiber.[13]

Certain traditional herbal remedies, like flaxseed, milled flax, and linseed, serve as excellent sources of fiber and can be beneficial in treating constipation during pregnancy. These are typically incorporated into liquids or food items, such as bread or muffins. However, it is important to note that there is insufficient evidence regarding the safety of these remedies during pregnancy.[14]

According to Longo et al., probiotics may have a positive impact on the overall bowel function by favorably altering the colonic flora.[15] A recent study conducted by The UC Davis School of Medicine has found that probiotics significantly improve symptoms associated with pregnancy, such as nausea, vomiting, and constipation.[16]

In addition, regular exercise in the form of walking, dancing, swimming, or cycling can improve digestion and alleviate bowel symptoms.[7] Laxatives are prescribed if dietary and lifestyle modifications fail to improve the symptoms.

Bulk-forming Agents

Bulk-forming agents such as psyllium, methylcellulose, and bran are among the agents of choice for initial therapy during pregnancy. These are not absorbed and do not produce malabsorption, so are considered safe for even long-term use in pregnancy.[17] These agents make the stool bulky and soft due to their high water-binding capacity. These are generally well tolerated and serious side effects are rare. Common adverse effects include bloating sensation, abdominal cramps, diarrhea, and nausea.[3]

Stool Softeners

Docusate sodium is considered safe and no teratogenic effect has been associated with its use during pregnancy. Since it is not absorbed from gastrointestinal tract, there are no known systemic side effects. Docusate is an anionic surfactant, which works by reducing the surface tension of the stool, allowing water to mix with stool, making it moist and easier to pass. The typical daily dosage ranges from 100 to 400 mg when taken orally, usually divided into multiple doses.

Lubricant Laxatives

Lubricant laxatives such as mineral oils work by coating the stool with a waterproof layer and hence retaining its moisture. This keeps the stool soft and smooth. Because the mineral oils are not absorbed from the gastrointestinal tract, there are no associated systemic side effects. The mineral oil may hamper absorption of fat-soluble vitamins so it is recommended to use it on an empty stomach. Common side effects include diarrhea, fecal urgency, anal irritation, and oily rectal discharge. Additionally, the safety of mineral oil for long-term use, particularly during pregnancy, is not well established, and its usage should be avoided unless strongly indicated.[18]

Osmotic Laxatives

The group of osmotic laxatives include lactulose, sorbitol, polyethylene glycol (PEG). These drugs act as hyperosmolar agents, causing increased water retention in the colonic lumen. Lactulose and PEG are poorly absorbed and do not appear to be associated with systemic adverse effects. The dosage for sorbitol and lactulose is 15–30 mL/day.[3,5]

Lactulose is still regarded as the treatment of choice for chronic constipation in pregnancy by The American Gastroenterology Association, The American Family Doctor's Association, RCOG, and FOGSI.

Additionally, Lactulose, owing to its prebiotic effect, can cause increased growth of endogenous bacteria that are potentially beneficial to the host like Lactobacilli, thereby indirectly reducing the strength of potentially more harmful urease producing bacteria. This can help maintain the integrity of the epithelial barrier and mucosal immune system, thereby maintaining intestinal homeostasis along with lasting relief from constipation.

Stimulant Laxatives

Stimulant laxatives, such as bisacodyl and senna, act on the intestinal mucosa, increasing water and electrolyte secretion. They also stimulate colonic peristalsis. While they may provide effective relief for constipation, their safety during pregnancy is not well established.[3] Some studies suggest a possible association with uterine contractions. Therefore, their use is generally limited to short durations and avoided during the first and third trimesters. Both senna and bisacodyl are not associated with any teratogenic or fetotoxic effect. Bisacodyl is classified under pregnancy category C. It can be administered orally in pill form at a dosage of 10–15 mg or as a 10-mg suppository rectally. Bisacodyl use may be associated with increased abdominal cramping compared to senna-containing laxatives.[3,5]

New Agents

New agents such as prucalopride, linaclotide, and lubiprostone have emerged for the management of chronic constipation, but their use during pregnancy requires careful consideration. Prucalopride stimulates the serotonin 5-HT4 receptor, altering colonic motility to facilitate defecation. While it is approved for chronic constipation in non-pregnant individuals, limited data exist on its use during pregnancy, and it is not recommended during this period or breastfeeding.[19] Linaclotide, a guanylate cyclase-C receptor agonist, is categorized as a pregnancy class C drug. Its approval is for the management of irritable bowel syndrome associated with constipation (IBS-C). Similarly, lubiprostone, a locally acting chloride channel 2 (ClC-2) activator, is approved for chronic idiopathic constipation. However, caution is advised during pregnancy and breastfeeding due to limited information on their safety. The decision to use these drugs should weigh potential benefits against potential risks to the fetus, and effective contraception is recommended for women of childbearing potential during treatment with prucalopride.[8,19]

Laxative to be Avoided During Pregnancy

Castor oil and sodium-containing osmotic agents are not recommended for pregnant women. Castor oil is contraindicated during pregnancy and has a pregnancy class X precaution. The use of sodium-containing laxatives, like phospho-soda, may result in systemic sodium and water retention, posing potential risks for pregnant women.[3,5]

Aloe also exhibits a laxative effect; however, due to a reported association with congenital malformations, the use of *aloe* is not recommended during pregnancy.[5]

Flowchart 1: Algorithm for the treatment of constipation in pregnancy.

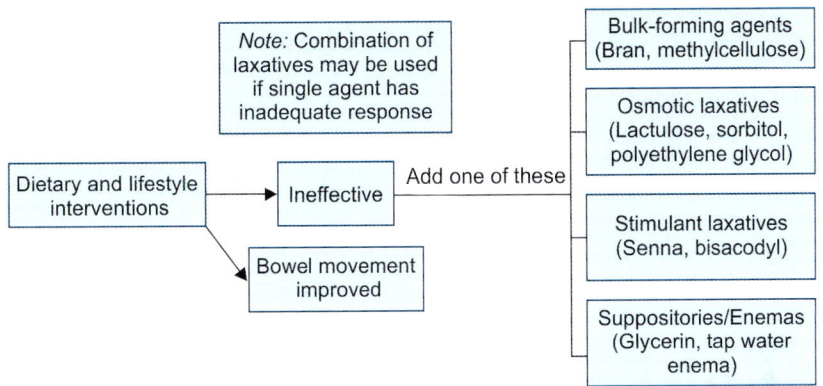

Enemas and Suppositories

Patients experiencing fecal loading or impaction may find relief through the use of glycerine suppositories, in conjunction with oral laxatives as needed. The UK Teratology Information Service suggests that glycerine suppositories can be utilized during pregnancy. The use of phosphate enemas during pregnancy and their potential for teratogenic effects lacks specific data in published studies, therefore, it is advisable to avoid their use during pregnancy.[8,20]

Discontinuation of Laxatives

The laxatives should be gradually stopped once regular bowel movements are achieved. The reduction in laxative dosage should be guided by the frequency and consistency of stools. Gradual withdrawal helps minimize the risk of needing to restart therapy for recurrent fecal loading. If a combination of laxatives is being used, it is advisable to stop one laxative at a time, with stimulant laxatives reduced first. Relapses are common, and they are managed by promptly increasing the laxative dose.[8]

■ CONCLUSION

Decisions regarding the treatment of constipation during pregnancy should prioritize concerns about safety. The initial approach to constipation management involves dietary and lifestyle modifications. If this proves ineffective, laxatives should be considered. Most of the patients can be managed with bulk-forming laxatives. Stimulant laxatives should be used with caution in patients not responding to safer alternatives **(Flowchart 1)**.

When red flag symptoms are present, such as refractory or worsening constipation, rectal bleeding, a known history of gastrointestinal disorders like inflammatory bowel disease, or a family history of colorectal cancer, a prompt referral to a gastroenterologist for detailed work-up is warranted.

■ REFERENCES

1. Jewell DJ, Young G. Interventions for treating constipation in pregnancy. Cochrane Database Syst Rev. 2001(2):CD001142.
2. Cullen G, O'Donoghue D. Constipation and pregnancy. Best Pract Res Clin Gastroenterol. 2007;21(5):807-18.
3. Trottier M, Erebara A, Bozzo P. Treating constipation during pregnancy. Can Fam Physician. 2012;58(8):836-8.
4. Bradley CS, Kennedy CM, Turcea AM, Rao SS, Nygaard IE. Constipation in pregnancy: prevalence, symptoms, and risk factors. Obstet Gynecol. 2007;110(6):1351-7.

5. Prather CM. Pregnancy-related constipation. Curr Gastroenterol Rep. 2004;6(5):402-4.
6. Mearin F, Lacy BE, Chang L, Chey WD, Lembo AJ, Simren M, et al. Bowel disorders. Gastroenterology. 2016;150(6):1393-407.
7. Derbyshire E, Davies J, Costarelli V, Dettmar P. Diet, physical inactivity and the prevalence of constipation throughout and after pregnancy. Matern Child Nutr. 2006;2(3):127-34.
8. Verghese TS, Futaba K, Latthe P. Constipation in pregnancy. The Obstetrician and Gynaecologist. 2015;17(20):111-5.
9. Gill RC, Bowes KL, Kingma YJ: Effect of progesterone on canine colonic smooth muscle. Gastroenterology. 1985;88:1941-7.
10. Ryan JP, Bhojwani A. Colonic transit in rats: effect of ovariectomy, sex steroid hormones, and pregnancy. Am J Physiol. 1986;251:G46-50.
11. Shin GH, Toto EL, Schey R. Pregnancy and postpartum bowel changes: constipation and fecal incontinence. Am J Gastroenterol. 2015;110(4):521-9; quiz 530.
12. Anderson AS, Whichelow MJ: Constipation during pregnancy: dietary fibre intake and the effect of fibre supplementation. Hum Nutr Appl Nutr. 1985;39:202-7.
13. Marlett JA, McBurney MI, Slavin JL. Position of the American Dietetic Association: health implications of dietary fiber. J Am Diet Assoc. 2002;102:993-1000.
14. Medicines and Healthcare Products Regulatory Agency. PAR; Linoforce Granules. THR 13668/0021. London: MHRA; 2001.
15. Longo SA, Moore RC, Canzoneri BJ, Robichaux A. Gastrointestinal conditions during pregnancy. Clin Colon Rectal Surg. 2010;23(2):80-9.
16. Liu AT, Chen S, Jena PK, Sheng L, Hu Y, Wan YY. Probiotics Improve Gastrointestinal Function and Life Quality in Pregnancy. Nutrients. 2021;13(11):3931.
17. Jick H, Holmes LB, Hunter JR, Madsen S, Stergachis A. First-trimester drug use and congenital disorders. JAMA. 1981;246(4):343-6.
18. Servey J, Chang J. Over-the-Counter Medications in Pregnancy. Am Fam Physician. 2014;90(8):548-55. Erratum in: Am Fam Physician. 2015;92(5):332.
19. National Institute for Health and Care Excellence. Prucalopride for the Treatment of Chronic Constipation in Women. Technology Appraisal Guidance [TA211]. London: NICE, 2010. [online] Available from: https://www.nice.org.uk/guidance/ta211 [Last accessed December, 2023].
20. UK Teratology Information Service. (2022). Treatment of Constipation in Pregnancy. [online] Available from: https://uktis.org/monographs/treatment-of-constipation-in-pregnancy/ [Last accessed December, 2023].

Index

Page numbers followed by *b* refer to box, *f* refer to figure, and *t* refer to table.

A

Abdominal distention, progressive 144
Abdominal pain 134
ABO blood group 93
  incompatibility 92
Achieve meticulous fluid balance 15
Acquired immunodeficiency syndrome 125, 127
  etiopathogenesis of 125
Activated partial thromboplastin time 10, 59
Acute kidney injury 76
  pregnancy-related 76
  reasons of 76*b*
Acute nephritic syndrome 79
Acute renal failure 68
  complication of 77
Acute respiratory distress syndrome 68, 119
  progression of 134
Adaptive immunity 73
Adenosine triphosphate 133
Adverse fetal outcomes 121
Alanine
  aminotransferase 110
  transaminase 9, 66
Albuterol metered dose inhaler 46
Albuterol nebulizer 46
Alloimmunized pregnancy, management of 92
Aloe 146
Aminophylline 46
Amnestic response 91
Amniocentesis 95
Amniotic fluid spectral analysis 95
Amoxicillin 115
Ampicillin plus gentamicin 116
Anal fissure, acute 144
Anemia 1, 3, 69
  causes of 1
  classification 1
  clinical features of 3
  diagnosis of 3
  effects of 2
  phases of 2
  reverse 4

Angiotensin-converting enzyme 60, 105
  receptors 133
Anorexia 144
Antenatal care 29
  regular assessment of 56
  regular structured 128
Antenatal complications 29*t*
Antenatal steroid use 137
Antepartum 2
  complications 29
  hemorrhage 93
  management principles 56
Anticoagulants 59
  use of 138
Antiepileptic drugs 83, 84
  classification of 84
  pharmacokinetics of 86
Antinuclear antibody 100
Antiphospholipid
  antibodies 14, 74, 102
  syndrome 100
Antiretroviral prophylaxis 130
Antiretroviral therapy, goals of 130
Antiretroviral treatment 127
  toxicity monitoring 128
Aorta, coarctation of 59
Aortic regurgitation 58
Aortic stenosis 58
Aortic valve area 61
Ascites, severe 68
Aspartate transaminase 9, 66
Aspirin 105
Asthma 42-44
  control 48
  test 45
  diagnosis of 43
  evaluation of 44
  exacerbation, acute 46
  management of 45
  relation of 44*t*
Asymptomatic bacteriuria 113, 115, 115*t*
Atonic postpartum hemorrhage 57
Atrial septal defect 58
Autism spectrum disorder 32
Autoimmune
  diseases, behavior of 73
  hepatitis 66

Azathioprine 67, 104, 105
Azotemia 79
Aztreonam 116

B

Bacterial infections, severe 126
Beclomethasone dipropionate 46
Betamethasone 138
Biliary cirrhosis, primary 64
Biophysical tests 24*t*
Bloating sensation 145
Blood
  disorder 1
  parameters 10
  pressure 52, 72
    raised 68
  transfusion 6
  urea nitrogen 79, 128
Body mass index 15, 18, 28, 29, 137
Bowel dysfunction 143
Bowel problems, history of 143
Brain 11
Breastfeeding 32, 111, 138
  exclusive 131
Brivaracetam 84
Budesonide 46
Bulk-forming agents 145

C

Calcineurin inhibitors 104, 105
Calcium 144
Carbamazepine 85-87
Carbon monoxides testing, capacity of lungs for 44
Cardiac arrhythmias 60
Cardiac disease 51*t*, 52
Cardiac dysfunction 29
Cardiac failure 2
Cardiac lesions, specific 54
Cardiac troponin 53
Cardiotocography 88
Cardiovascular disease 50, 52, 54*t*
  clinical indicators of 52*t*
  prevalence of 51*f*
Carpreg score 60*t*, 61*t*
Cefepime 116
Cefpodoxime 115
Ceftriaxone 116

Centers for Disease Control and
    Prevention 1, 139
  analysis 134
Central nervous system 85, 119, 120
Cephalexin 115
Cerebral edema retinal
    detachment 68
Cesarean
  delivery, incidence of 135
  section 31
Chest
  diameter 43
  X-ray 52
Chlamydia 128
  trachomatis 115
Cholelithiasis 64, 67
Chorea 101
Chorionic
    somatomammotropin 16
Chronic kidney disease 72
Chronic obstructive pulmonary
    disease 42
Cirrhosis 66
Colonic stricture 144
Complete blood count 122
Congenital abnormalities 17
Constipation 143, 143*b*
  causes of 144*b*
  chronic 143*b*
  development of 144
  pregnancy-related 143, 144
  prevalence of functional 143
Contraception 86
Convulsion 12, 12*t*
Coombs test, indirect 93
Coronary artery
  bypass grafting 60
  diseases 60
Coronavirus disease-2019
    (COVID-19) 139, 139*t*
  vaccination 135
  vaccine 136
Cortical necrosis, acute 77
Corticosteroids 104
Cotrimoxazole preventive
    therapy 128
Covaxin 136
Covishield 136
Cromolyn 46
Cyclophosphamide 103, 105
Cyclosporine 67, 105
Cystitis 115
  acute 113
Cytomegalovirus 96
  infection, congenital 68

D

Dehydration 144
Delivery
  estimated date of 24, 56
  mode of 111
  route of 24
  timing of 24, 31
Dengue 118-120, 120*b*, 121
  diagnosis of 120
  fever 120, 122
    clinical phases of 119*b*
  hemorrhagic fever 119
  management of 121
    protocols of 122
  severe 120
  shock syndrome 119
  virus, pathophysiology of 119*f*
Deoxyribonucleic acid 65, 110
  cell-free 93
  double-stranded 100
Diabetes mellitus 16, 17*t*, 18, 51*f*
  type 1 19
  type 2 19
Diabetic nephropathy 78
Diaphragm 43
Diarrhea 145
Dietary advice 4
Dietary modification 144
Dietary therapy 21
Digital fecal evacuation 144
Direct agglutinin test 97
Disodium cromoglycate 46
Disseminated intravascular
    coagulation 67, 69, 119,
    120
Dolutegravir 128, 130
Dysfunctional labor 2

E

Echocardiography 53
Eclampsia 11, 12*t*, 14, 76
  intercurrent 11
Edema, triple 98
Eisenmenger syndrome 56, 59
Electrocardiogram 52
Encephalitis 119
Endocrine system 10
End-organ damage,
    mechanism of 10
Endothelial cells 10
Enemas 147
Enzyme-linked immunosorbent
    assay 120

Epilepsy 83, 86, 87
  classification of 83
Erythroblastosis fetalis 91
Erythrocyte sedimentation
    rate 100
Escherichia coli 114
Eslicarbazepine 84, 86
Estrogen 16, 114
Everolimus 67
Exercise 144
  stress test 53
Extracorporeal membrane
    oxygenation 134, 139
Extractable nuclear antigens 100

F

Fasting glucose, impaired 25
Fasting plasma glucose 18
Fatty liver disease, nonalcoholic 29
Febrile phase 119
Fecal impaction 144
Feeding, exclusive replacement
    131
Fentanyl 138
Fetal anemia 91
  severe 96
  severity of 94
Fetal anomaly, targeted
    imaging for 87
Fetal blood sampling 95
Fetal brain development 37
Fetal complications 12*t*
Fetal effects 38, 39
Fetal growth
  assessment 24
  restriction 9
Fetal hemoglobin 93
Fetal hyperbilirubinemia 91
Fetal hyperglycemia leads 17
Fetal monitoring 102
Fetal red blood cell 94
Fetal surveillance 48
  tests 102
Fetomaternal hemorrhage 93
  causes of 90*b*
  insufficient amount of 89
Fetotoxic effect 146
Fetus 3
Flavivirus 118, 120
Fluid electrolyte levels 10
Flunisolide 46
Fluticasone propionate 46
Folate deficiency 6
Food and Drug Administration 86

Forced vital capacity 43
Fosphenytoin 84
Functional residual capacity 133

G

Gabapentin 84
Gallstones 64, 67
Gaseous distention 145
Gastroesophageal reflux
　　disease 44
Gastrointestinal tract 143
Gastrointestinal transit 144
Gestational age, large for 17, 22
Gestational diabetes mellitus 16,
　　18, 23*t*, 128
　consequences of 17
　management of 22
　prevention of 26
　screening 128
Gestational hypertension 74
Gestational weight gain 29
Glomerular filtration rate 72, 73
Glomerulonephritis 79
　acute 79
Glyburide 22
Glycemic control
　monitoring 23
　target 23
Glycerine 147
Goodpasture syndrome 79
Grandmother erythrocytes 92
Grandmother theory 91
Graves' disease 38
Gravid uterus 144
Great artery, transposition of 17
Guanylate cyclase-C receptor
　　agonist 146

H

Hashimoto thyroiditis 39
Heart
　rate 52
　transplantation 60
Heart block
　complete 101
　congenital 105
Heart disease 50, 61
　classification of functional 53
　congenital 58
　diagnosis of 51
Hemodynamics index 73*t*
Hemoglobin 139
　low levels of 1

Hemoglobinopathy 1
Hemolysis 69
　elevated liver enzyme, and low
　　　platelet count 64, 69, 76
　syndrome 13*t*, 68, 76
Hemolytic anemia, congenital 90
Hemolytic disease 89
Hemolytic jaundice 64
Hemolytic uremic syndrome 68, 69
Hemorrhagic blood loss
　acute 1
　chronic 1
Heparin, unfractionated 59, 105
Hepatitis
　A virus 64
　B
　　chronic 110
　　E antigen 110
　　signs of acute 109
　　surface antigen, serological
　　　　detection of 65
　　symptoms of acute 109
　　vaccine 65
　B infection 108
　　vertical transmission of 110
　B virus 65, 108, 110
　　infection 110*t*
　C virus 65
　E virus 65
Hepatosplenomegaly 91
Histocompatibility complex,
　　maternal major 10
Hodgkin's disease 1
Human chorionic gonadotropin,
　　high levels of 37
Human immunodeficiency virus
　　125-127, 130, 131
　infection
　　signs of 126
　　symptoms of 126
　　transmission, risk of 127*t*
Hydralazine 11, 104, 105
Hydrops fetalis 89, 91, 97
Hydroxychloroquine 104
　effects of 105
Hypercalcemia 144
Hyperemesis gravidarum 68
　severe 64
Hyperglycemia, prevalence of 16
Hypertension 29, 51
　chronic 13, 74
　control of 14
　portal 66
　pregnancy-induced 79
　risk of chronic 67

Hypertensive disorder 8, 30, 74, 135
　of pregnancy,
　　classification of 8
Hyperthyroidism 37, 38
　subclinical 38
　symptoms of 38*t*
　treatment of overt 38
Hyperventilation syndrome 44
Hypoglycemia 69
Hypothyroidism 38, 39, 144
　signs of 39*t*
　subclinical 39
　symptoms of 39*t*
　treatment of overt 39

I

Icterus gravis neonatorum 90
Idiopathic hypertrophic subaortic
　　stenosis 59
Immune
　complexes, deposition of 99
　cytotrophoblastic-mediated
　　cytotrophoblastic
　　cell 10
　hydrops 91
Immunization, active 65
Immunoglobulin G,
　role of 135
　M 120, 135
In vitro fertilization 10
Infections 1
Inhaled corticosteroids 46
Innate immunity 73
Insulin
　lispro 21
　pump 21
　therapy 21, 23
Integrase inhibitor 130
Intelligence quotient 87
Intensive care unit 134, 139
Intensive coronary care unit 122
Interleukin 139
International Diabetes
　　Federation 16
International Federation of
　　Gynecology and
　　Obstetrics 18
International League Against
　　Epilepsy 84
Intrapartum
　complications 30, 30*t*
　management
　　glycemic 25
　　principles 56

Intraperitoneal transfusion 96
Intrauterine
    contraceptive device 58
    exposure 16
    fetal death 93
    growth restriction 79, 101, 102
    transfusion 96
Intravascular transfusion 96
Invasive ventilation 134
Iron 144
    dextran 5
    requirement 2
    sucrose complex 5
    supplements 144
Iron deficiency
    anemia 2
        etiology of 2
    prevention of 4
Irritable bowel syndrome 146

J

Jaundice 69
    differential diagnosis of 69t
Jugular venous pressure 3, 52

K

Kaposi's sarcoma 126
Kell alloimmunization 92
Kidneys 10
Klebsiella pneumoniae 114
Kleihauer–Betke test 93
Labetalol 11
    nifedipine 104

L

Lacosamide 84
Lactulose 145, 146
Lamivudine 128
Lamotrigine 84, 85
Laxatives
    discontinuation of 147
    lubricant 145
    osmotic 145, 146
    stimulant 146
Left ventricular ejection
        fraction 61
Leukotriene 46
    antagonists 46
Levetiracetam 84, 85
Life-threatening pneumonia
        infection 134

Linaclotide 146
Lithotomy position 57
Liver 11
    diseases 64
        classification of 64t
    function tests 65
    transplant 67
Low potency 46
Low-birth-weight 119
Low-molecular-weight heparin 60
Lung capacity 42
Lupus
    anticoagulant 102
    development of 99
    glomerulonephritis 79
    nephritis 103

M

Macrocytic anemias 3
Marfan's syndrome 56, 59
Mast cell stabilizers 46
Maternal complications 12t
Maternal diabetes 20
Maternal fetal
    management 16, 50
    metabolism 16
Maternal hyperglycemia leads 17
Maternal monitoring 102
Maternal obesity 28
Medical nutrition therapy 22, 23
Medical termination of
        pregnancy 128
Membrane
    premature rupture of 67
    proliferative
        glomerulonephritis 79
Menstrual irregularities 28
Metformin 22, 23
Methotrexate 105
Methylcellulose 145
Methyldopa 11, 104, 105
Methylergonovine 138
Methylprednisolone 47
Microcytic anemias 3
Microthrombosis 11
Midazolam 138
Middle cerebral artery-peak
        systolic velocity 95
Mirror syndrome 98
Mitral regurgitation 58
Mitral stenosis 58
Molnupiravir 137, 138
Mometasone furoate 46
Monoclonal antibodies 136

Motilin 144
Multiple gestation 93
Myocarditis 119

N

Nasal cannula, high-flow 139
National AIDS control
        organisation 130
National AIDS control
        programme 125
National Institute for Health
        and Care Excellence
        guidelines 30
National Institute of Virology 136
Natriuretic peptides 53
Nausea 144, 145
Neonatal intensive care
        unit 15, 25, 31
Newborn care, immediate 129
Nifedipine 11, 105, 138
Nitric oxide, fractional exhaled 45
Nitrofurantoin 115
Nitroglycerine 11
Nonfluorinated systemic steroids 46
Nonsteroidal anti-inflammatory
        drugs 64, 104, 122

O

Obesity 28, 30, 32, 51
    classification of 28t
    epidemic 16
    general consideration 28
    management of 28
Obstetric anesthesia
        principles 57
Obstructive sleep apnea 29, 52
Oral antimicrobial agents 115
Oral contraceptive failure 29
Oral hypoglycemic agent 22
Oral iron therapy 5
Oxcarbamazepine 84-86
Oxidative stress hypothesis 10

P

Parenteral iron therapy 5
Patchy cortical necrosis 77
Patent ductus arteriosus 17, 59
Paxlovid, use of 138
Peak expiratory flow 46
Peptide hormones 16
Periconceptional counseling 103
Periodic fetal biophysical testing 24

Peripartum cardiomyopathy 58
Persistent infections 116
Personal protective equipment 137
Phenobarbital 84, 86
Phenytoin 84, 86
Phospho-soda 146
Physiological anemia 1
Physiological hydronephrosis 73
Piperacillin 116
Placenta 11
Placental changes 9
Placental steroid 16
Plasma ferritin concentrations 3
Pleural effusion 68
Polycystic ovary syndrome 22
Polyethylene glycol 145
Postpartum
  care 25
  complications 31, 31t
  depression 40
  hemorrhage, risk of 32
  management 31, 111
    principles 57
  obstetric problems 57
  period 15
  surveillance 103
  thyroiditis 40
Postprandial hyperglycemia 17
Poststreptococcal
    glomerulonephritis 79
Postural hypotension 3
Preconception counseling 54, 86
Prediabetes 20
Preeclampsia 8-10, 12t, 14, 67, 75,
    75t, 76, 79, 101, 103
  classification of 9t
  early-onset 9
  first trimester screening for 13
  late-onset 9
  management of 14, 75
  pathogenesis of 9
  prevention of 13
  risk factors for 8t
  screening of 13
  signs of 75
Pregabalin 84, 86
Pregestational diabetes 29
Pregnancy 1, 2, 9, 12, 13, 16, 28,
    37-40, 43-45, 50, 50t,
    52, 52t, 61, 64, 64t, 67,
    69t, 72, 72t, 76b, 77, 83,
    86, 87, 99, 101, 108, 113,
    114, 118, 120-122, 125,
    126, 133, 135, 137, 138
  acute fatty liver of 64, 67, 69

  care delivery location 54
  complication of 101
  effects of 100
  hypertensive disorders of 8,
    74, 135
  intrahepatic cholestasis of 66
  loss 90
  uncomplicated 73t
Pregnancy-related disorders,
    pathogenesis of 74
Prenatal obstetric management 24
Prepregnancy 28
  management 20
Preterm birth 101
Preterm delivery 67
Pretransfusion sample 96
Primidone 86
Progesterone 16, 114, 144
Prophylactic platelet
    transfusion 122
Prosthetic valves 59
Proteinuria 29, 73
Proteus mirabilis 114
Prucalopride stimulates 146
Psyllium 145
Pulmonary edema 68
Pulmonary embolism 44
Pulmonary endothelial cell
    dysfunction 134
Pulmonary hypertension 59
  primary 56
Pulmonary stenosis 59
Pulse oximetry 45
Pus cells 116
Pyelonephritis 116t
  acute 113, 115
  treatment regimens for 116

R

Red cell alloimmunization 89, 90b
Renal biopsy 103
Renal complications 77
Renal disease
  chronic 77
  mild 77
  severe 77
Renal disorders 72
Renal failure, chronic 77
Renal function tests 116
Renal insufficiency 77
Renal plasma flow 73
Respiratory alkalemia,
    compensatory 133
Respiratory distress syndrome 116

Respiratory rate 52
Respiratory system 43t
Rh alloimmunization 89
  epidemiology 89
  genetics 89
  pathophysiology 90
Rh D alloimmunization,
    prevention of 94
Rh isoimmunization
  fetal effects of 90
  maternal effects of 91
Rhesus
  blood type 92
  factor 89
Ribonucleic acid virus 64, 65
  single stranded 118, 133
Right ventricular systolic
    pressure 61
Rufinamide 84

S

SARS-CoV-2 133
  infection 137, 138, 140
    effects of 134
    mother-to-child
      transmission of 135
    prevention of 135
  monoclonal antibodies 136
  presentation of 134
  vaccination against 135
  virus 133
Sclerosing cholangitis, primary 64
Semi allogeneic fetus,
    growth of 133
Seminal priming 10
Sepsis 68
Serological methods 120
Serum
  alkaline phosphatase 66
  anti-hepatitis A virus 64
  free thyroxine levels 37
Sexually transmitted infection 127
Sickle cell disease 1
Sirolimus 67
Sodium
  containing osmotic agents 146
  nitroprusside 11
Soluble endoglin
    proinflammatory
      cytokine 10
Sorbitol 145, 146
Spirometry 44
Spontaneous coronary artery
    dissection 60

Index

Sputnik V 136
Status eclampticus 11
Steroid therapy, long-term 104
Stool softeners 145
Streptococcal infection, group B 113
Streptococcus faecalis 114
Sudden unexpected death 87
Sulfamethoxazole 129
Sustainable development growth 131
Systemic connective tissue disease, chronic 99
Systemic lupus erythematosus 14, 74, 78, 99, 102
  clinical features 99
  diagnosis 100
  effects of 101
  incidence 99
  pathogenesis 99
  preconception evaluation 99
  pregnancy 102t, 104t

T

Tachypnea 3
Tacrolimus 67, 105
Tazobactam 116
Tenofovir 128
Teratogenic effect 146
Tetralogy of Fallot 59
Thalassemia 1
Thrombocyte 69
Thrombocytopenia 101
Thrombosed hemorrhoids 144
Thrombosis 101
Thrombotic thrombocytopenic purpura 68, 69
Thyroid
  cancer 40
  disease 39
  disorder 37, 39

  function 37, 40
  nodule 40
Thyroid storm 40
  clinical features of 40t
  signs of 40
  symptoms of 40
Thyroid-stimulating hormone, level of 37
Thyrotoxic heart failure 40
Tiagabine 84
Tocolytics 144
Topiramate 84, 86
Tranexamic acid 138
Transaminase 69
Transcriptase-polymerase chain reaction, reverse 120
Transplacental transmission 135
Trichomonas 128
Tricuspid valve diseases 58
Trimethoprim 129
Trophoblast
  debris 10
  invasion 74
Tuberculosis 64, 126
Tubular necrosis, acute 76

U

Ultrasound assessment 95
Upper respiratory tract 43
Urethritis 115
Urinary tract infection 1, 13
  bacteriology 114
  epidemiology 113
  etiopathogenesis 114
  management 116
  screening of 114
  signs 114
  symptoms 114
Urine 69
Ursodeoxycholic acid 66

Uteroplacental insufficiency 11
Uterus, subinvolution of 3

V

Vaccination assessment 128
Vaginal birth after cesarean 30
Valproate 85, 87
  extent of 87
Valvular heart diseases 58
Vascular endothelial growth factor 10
Vasculitis 99
Vasectomy 57
Ventricular septal defect 17, 58
Vigabatrin 84
Viral hepatitis 64
  screening 128
Viral infection 108
Viral load measurement 128
Vital capacity 43
Vitamin, fat-soluble 145
Vomiting 144

W

Warfarin 60
Weight gain 29t

Y

Yellow fever 120

Z

Zafirlukast 46
Zahara prediction score 60, 61t
Zika virus 120
Zileuton theophylline 46
Zonisamide 84